SpringerBriefs in Computer Science

SpringerBriefs present concise summaries of cutting-edge research and practical applications across a wide spectrum of fields. Featuring compact volumes of 50 to 125 pages, the series covers a range of content from professional to academic.

Typical topics might include:

- A timely report of state-of-the art analytical techniques
- A bridge between new research results, as published in journal articles, and a contextual literature review
- A snapshot of a hot or emerging topic
- An in-depth case study or clinical example
- A presentation of core concepts that students must understand in order to make independent contributions

Briefs allow authors to present their ideas and readers to absorb them with minimal time investment. Briefs will be published as part of Springer's eBook collection, with millions of users worldwide. In addition, Briefs will be available for individual print and electronic purchase. Briefs are characterized by fast, global electronic dissemination, standard publishing contracts, easy-to-use manuscript preparation and formatting guidelines, and expedited production schedules. We aim for publication 8–12 weeks after acceptance. Both solicited and unsolicited manuscripts are considered for publication in this series.

**Indexing: This series is indexed in Scopus, Ei-Compendex, and zbMATH **

Asma Channa · Nirvana Popescu

Deep Learning in Smart eHealth Systems

Evaluation Leveraging for Parkinson's Disease

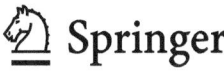 Springer

Asma Channa 🆔
Department of Computer Science
Politehnica University of Bucharest
Bucharest, Romania

Nirvana Popescu 🆔
Department of Computer Science
Politehnica University of Bucharest
Bucharest, Romania

ISSN 2191-5768   ISSN 2191-5776   (electronic)
SpringerBriefs in Computer Science
ISBN 978-3-031-45002-0   ISBN 978-3-031-45003-7   (eBook)
https://doi.org/10.1007/978-3-031-45003-7

This Springer imprint is published by the registered company Springer Nature Switzerland AG
The registered company address is: Gewerbestrasse 11, 6330 Cham, Switzerland

Paper in this product is recyclable.

Preface

Motor deterioration is commonly observed in individuals with neurocognitive disorders (NCDs), significantly impacting their overall quality of life. One prominent form of NCD is Parkinson's Disease (PD), typically developing after the age of 60. Traditional clinical assessment of PD relies on subjective rating scales, which are time-consuming and prone to inaccuracies.

In recent years, significant advancements have been made in automating the diagnosis and severity assessment of Parkinson's disease. These approaches can be broadly categorized into two types: those utilizing hand-crafted features and classifiers based on standard instructions, and those employing fully automated methods powered by deep learning (DL). The former involves manually selecting specific features as input for classifiers, with no modifications to the classifiers during training. The latter focuses on fully automated techniques that leverage DL, allowing for parameter adjustments to accommodate diverse training data scenarios. DL eliminates the need for manual feature engineering and has proven highly adaptable in overcoming medical diagnostic challenges associated with PD.

This book aims to provide neurologists with reliable wearable devices for objectively assessing motor impairments in individuals with PD. To achieve this objective, a novel framework has been developed specifically for evaluating motor deficits in the upper extremities of PD patients. The proposed system integrates wearable technology, DL techniques, and cloud computing.

As part of this system, a compact wearable bracelet has been designed to continuously collect movement-related data. This data is then transmitted to a smartphone using Bluetooth Low Energy and processed through a mobile application serving as the user interface. The system utilizes a wireless network to connect to the MS Azure cloud, where the ServiceNow platform is employed as a web application. Movement data is stored in a database for further analysis. To address potential biases stemming from imbalanced data distribution, resampling techniques are applied, improving the accuracy of tremor severity estimation and ensuring more precise assessments.

The primary audience for this book consists of professionals seeking to enhance their proficiency in these technologies. However, the content is designed to cater to a diverse range of readers, with a specific focus on three target groups. One group comprises researchers interested in exploring the application of DL and wearable technology for assessing PD patients. Another target audience includes PD patients and practitioners who may not possess a background in DL or wearable computing but wish to swiftly acquire the necessary knowledge and effectively utilize medical wearables when needed.

Overall, this book endeavors to provide valuable insights and practical guidance to empower professionals, researchers, and individuals involved in the assessment and management of PD using innovative technological approaches.

Bucharest, Romania   Asma Channa
June 2023   Nirvana Popescu

Acknowledgements

First and foremost, we would like to thank Prof. Giuseppe Ruggeri from Mediterranea University of Reggio Calabria for extensive feedback and discussions that significantly improved this book. Additionally, we express our deep appreciation to Rares-Cristian Ifrim, prof. Decebal Popescu, Dr. Nadia Mammone, and Prof. Antonio Iera for their invaluable guidance, support, and mentorship throughout our research work.

As the authors, we sincerely acknowledge the funding received from the European Union's Horizon 2020 Research and Innovation program, granted under the Marie Skłodowska Curie grant agreement No. 813278 (A-WEAR: A network for dynamic wearable applications with privacy constraints, http://www.a-wear.eu/). Moreover, this work also received partial support from a grant provided by the Romanian National Authority for Scientific Research and Innovation, UEFISCDI project PNIII-P3-3.6-H2020-2020-0124.

Contents

Acronyms

NCDs	Neurocognitive Disorders
PD	Parkinson's Disease
FoG	Freezing of Gait
QoL	Quality of Life
BLE	Bluetooth Low Energy
DL	Deep Learning
L-dope	Levodopa
DLAs	Daily life Activities
ML	Machine Learning
HMM	Hidden Markov Model
SVM	Support Vector Machine
CWT	Continuous Wavelet Transform
IoT	Internet of Things
CNN	Convolutional Neural Network
DFA	Detrended Fluctuation Analysis
UI	User Interface

Chapter 1
Unraveling Parkinson's Disease: Diagnostic Challenges and Severity Assessment

Abstract Parkinson's Disease (PD) presents diagnostic complexities primarily reliant on subjective clinical assessments and the absence of definitive biomarkers. This chapter delves into the multifaceted diagnostic challenges associated with PD, including the heterogeneous progression of the disease, patient-reported biases, and the influence of medication. To evaluate disease severity, various rating scales like UPDRS and the Hoehn and Yahr scale are employed, though they have inherent limitations. Ongoing research efforts are dedicated to establishing more objective evaluation techniques leveraging wearable sensors and advanced imaging modalities. These advancements aim to enhance the precision of PD severity assessment, enabling the tailoring of personalized management strategies. Additionally, the chapter underscores the significance of distinguishing PD from conditions with similar symptomatology to prevent misdiagnosis, ultimately leading to improved patient outcomes and an elevated quality of life.

1.1 Introduction

Parkinson's disease (PD) is a chronic and progressive disorder that primarily affects the movement control centers of the brain. First described by Dr. James Parkinson in 1817 [1], it is characterized by both motor and non-motor symptoms. The prevalence rate of PD is approximately 10 million worldwide [2], with a higher incidence in men. In the United Kingdom alone, around 60,000 people are diagnosed with PD each year before the age of 50 [3], and the estimated rate is expected to double by 2030 [4].

Motor symptoms of PD include tremors, slowness of movement, stiffness, and balance problems, while non-motor symptoms encompass mental and behavioral changes, sleep disorders, hallucinations, sudden , and fatigue. Motor symptoms tend to dominate and worsen as the disease progresses, although the severity and progression can vary from person to person.

Currently, the diagnosis of PD relies primarily on clinical assessment and neurological evaluation, often utilizing the MDS-UPDRS (Movement Disorder Society-sponsored Unified Parkinson's Disease Rating Scale) [5]. Section 1.3 of the MDS-

UPDRS specifically focuses on evaluating motor impairment through standardized activities. Neurologists assign a score ranging from 0 (no motor symptoms) to 4 (severe motor symptoms) for each test, and the cumulative scores determine the patient's overall evaluation. However, this assessment method presents several challenges. Firstly, it is influenced by the patient's condition at the time of evaluation, which can vary. Additionally, the subjectivity of the evaluating clinicians introduces inter-rater variability, leading to potential inconsistencies in the assessment [6].

Addressing these challenges and developing more objective measures for assessing the severity of PD is crucial for accurate diagnosis and effective management of the disease.

1.2 Symptoms of Parkinson's Disease

The manifestations and indications of PD exhibit variability from person to person. Moreover, initial symptoms may appear subtle and go unnoticed. Typically, these signs initially manifest on a single side of the body and tend to remain more pronounced on that side, even as they progressively affect both limbs.

- **Tremors**: The initial limb to exhibit rhythmic shaking or tremor [7] is commonly one of the five fingers or the entire hand. Patients often notice trembling when they move their index finger and thumb. Similarly, the patient's hand skeleton might tremble while at rest. Interestingly, when the patient is focused on a task, the intensity of shaking can decrease. There are three distinct categories of tremors, each characterized by specific frequency ranges: Resting Tremor (RT) generally falls within the frequency range of 3–6 Hz, Postural tremor occurs between 6 and 9 Hz, and Kinetic tremor manifests in the frequency range of 9–12 Hz.
- **Bradykinesia (decelerate movement)**: Over time, PD has the potential to induce a gradual reduction in movement speed, posing challenges for everyday tasks that require precise timing. Consequently, the act of walking may involve shorter steps, making it difficult to rise from a sofa or perform actions with extended intervals. During walking, the patient might experience shuffling or dragging of the feet. This symptom is recognized as a fundamental characteristic of PD and is prevalent in approximately 80–90% of individuals with PD.
- **Rigidity**: In individuals with PD, muscle contractions can potentially occur in various parts of the body. Additionally, there is a likelihood of limited range of motion and discomfort due to the muscles becoming tense [8].
- **Freezing of Gait (FoG)**: is a common issue associated with PD. As per its definition, FoG refers to episodes of temporary cessation or significant reduction in the forward movement of the feet despite the intention to walk [9], and it's linked to an increased risk of falls. Recent studies have characterized FOG as a "sudden disruption of locomotor network dynamics" [10]. This phenomenon is often triggered by heightened cognitive demands, such as multitasking, or stressful sit-

uations. Measuring FOG in clinical settings presents challenges, as it can subside when the individual concentrates more on their walking pattern.

- **Posture and Balance Impairment**: This symptom emerges as a debilitating condition primarily in the later stages of the disease. Postural instability arises due to the absence of effective postural reflexes, causing individuals to struggle in maintaining a stable and balanced posture. This challenge becomes particularly evident during transitions, such as standing up, turning, or maneuvering while walking [11]. People with postural instability are at a heightened risk of falls, as they struggle to sustain an upright position. Earlier research indicates that approximately 60.5% of PD patients experienced at least one fall, while 39% encountered recurrent falls, averaging 20.8 falls per individual per year [11].

In clinical series, the occurrence of RT in patients with PD has been reported to be 90%, while in postmortem series, it has been reported to range from 76 to 100% [12]. The degree of tremor serves is a crucial indicator of PD severity and progression, aiding in the assessment of treatment effectiveness. The National Institute of Health (NIH) states that RT is the most common and readily identifiable symptom. It manifests as rhythmic, involuntary, and alternating movements primarily observed in the supported and relaxed upper and lower limbs, particularly in the hands. Hence, our proposed system revolves around the design of a tremor monitoring system, which could serve as a crucial marker for diagnosing PD and assessing its severity.

1.3 Clinical Diagnosis and Assessment Methods

Diagnosing PD does not rely on a specific test. Instead, PD is a diagnosis made through clinical evaluation, as depicted in Fig. 1.1, which outlines the entire PD assessment procedure. A neurologist evaluates PD patients by delving into their clinical history, reviewing their symptoms, and conducting a comprehensive neurological and physical examination.

The following numbered list presents the typical questions posed by neurologists during the process of diagnosing PD:

1. What sorts of side effects do you have?
2. When did these symptoms initially manifest, and how long have you been experiencing them?
3. Have there been any changes in the presentation of your symptoms?
4. Are you currently or have you previously been afflicted by any medical conditions or illnesses?
5. Are you currently taking any medications, including over-the-counter drugs?
6. Have any members of your family been diagnosed with certain medical conditions? Specifically, have any family members ever exhibited similar symptoms?
7. Have you ever had an allergic reaction to a medication? If so, could you provide the name of that medication?

Computer tomography (CT) and magnetic resonance imaging (MRI) scans of recognized quality are employed not only for detecting the possibility of PD but also for identifying various brain disorders such as cerebrovascular conditions and brain tumors. There is not a specific singular lab test or imaging procedure exclusively designed for diagnosing PD. To either confirm a PD diagnosis or explore other medical conditions that might resemble PD, specific methodologies like brain MRI, a dopamine transporter scan (DAT scan), or blood tests can be employed.

The doctor might recommend a specialized single-photon emission computerized tomography (SPECT) scan, known as a DAT scan, to assess the functionality of dopamine transporters (DAT). These proteins facilitate the recycling of dopamine, a neurotransmitter responsible for transmitting signals in the brain. The DAT scan is capable of distinguishing between conditions like PD and dementia with Lewy bodies (DLB) by visualizing the DAT's activity. While this can aid in strengthening the suspicion of PD, the ultimate accurate diagnosis is primarily determined by the symptoms and thorough neurological examination. However, it is important to note that not all individuals require a DAT scan.

Levodopa (L-dopa) stands as the benchmark treatment for addressing PD. A positive diagnosis of Parkinson's is often established when there is an improvement in motor symptoms upon administration of L-dopa. These diagnostic tests can be conducted multiple times to ensure a conclusive determination of whether a patient is indeed suffering from PD.

Frequently, medical professionals encounter challenges in accurately diagnosing PD and may sometimes associate it with other conditions that share similar symptoms. Diseases that exhibit symptom similarities to PD include:

1. **Parkinson's misdiagnosis: Arthritis**
   Misdiagnosing arthritis is not entirely implausible. Arthritis also presents symptoms like stiffness, restricted joint mobility, and joint discomfort. Consequently, the initial phases of PD often bear a strong resemblance to arthritis.
2. **Parkinson's misdiagnosis: General aging**
   It can be challenging to feel adequately acknowledged when your doctor assesses your symptoms and attributes them solely to the process of aging. While it is true that everyone experiences a natural decline in physical mobility as they grow older, it is important to recognize that Parkinson's has a more pronounced impact on both the physical and cognitive aspects of a person's well-being than the typical effects of aging.
3. **Parkinson's misdiagnosis: Huntington's disease**
   Huntington's disease leads to the degeneration of brain cells. Possible symptoms encompass clumsiness, insomnia, tiredness, and a decline in physical coordination. Since Huntington's disease often results in challenges with walking, it could indeed be a plausible diagnosis for an individual who is exhibiting symptoms resembling those of PD.
4. **Parkinson's misdiagnosis: Thyroid issues**
   Thyroid disorders can induce muscle weakness, leading to fatigue, discomfort, stiffness, and joint pain. The initial phases of PD may bear similarities to thyroid-

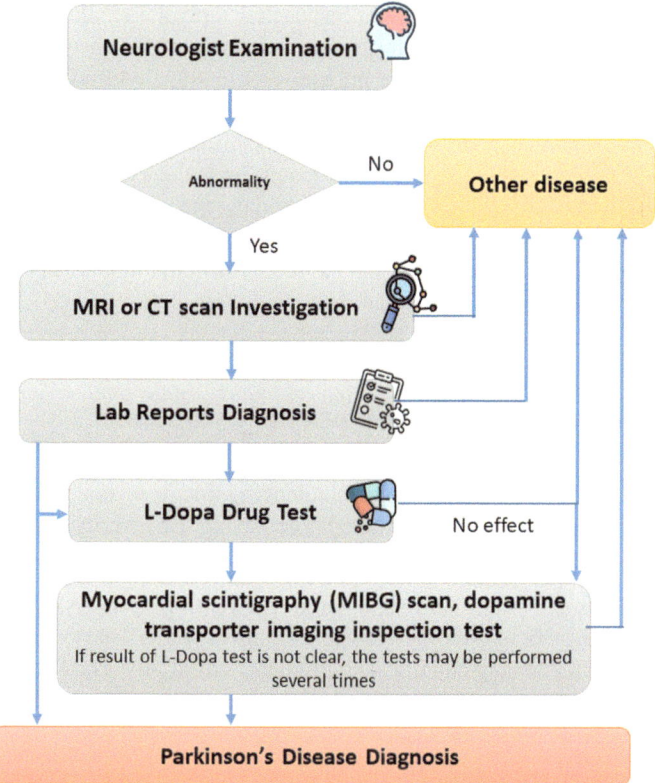

Fig. 1.1 Diagnosis of PD in a clinical setting

related concerns. Nonetheless, as patients become more acquainted with their own symptoms and gather insights over time, they can provide a more comprehensive perspective, aiding in the diagnostic process.

5. **Parkinson's misdiagnosis: Ankylosing spondylitis**
   Ankylosing spondylitis falls under the category of arthritis that leads to spinal rigidity and often hampers mobility. While some symptoms of ankylosing spondylitis overlap with PD, the latter presents a diverse array of additional symptoms. The journey towards an accurate diagnosis gains clarity as more distinct symptoms emerge.

Through the preceding discourse, the profound susceptibility of PD to significant misdiagnosis becomes unmistakably apparent, a predicament that frequently intertwines it with various other medical conditions. In light of this, the imperativeness of resilient apparatuses and methodologies emerges as a paramount factor in effectively distinguishing PD from its medical counterparts, thus mitigating the occurrences of misguided diagnoses.

Delving into the realm of technical intricacies, a pivotal challenge arises in the realm of prioritizing the seamless integration of Internet of Things (IoT) based wearables and the seamless automation of intricate processing algorithms. This endeavor holds the potential to establish an unyielding framework that can be effortlessly adopted by both medical practitioners and the Parkinson's patient cohort. The conceptualization and implementation of such an avant-garde device designed for in-home utilization could herald a transformative epoch in the management of PD. This innovation, extending its benefits not solely to patients but also amplifying the efficacy of healthcare systems, serves to fortify the realm of home monitoring capabilities, concurrently empowering patients and their caregivers alike.

1.4 Challenges in Finding Severity of Symptoms

Determining the severity of PD can be challenging due to several factors. Here are some of the common challenges involved in assessing the severity of PD:

1. **Subjectivity of Symptoms**

   PD symptoms can vary significantly from person to person. Symptoms such as tremors, rigidity, bradykinesia (slowness of movement), and postural instability can fluctuate in intensity and impact individuals differently. The subjective nature of these symptoms can make it challenging to objectively measure disease severity.

2. **Lack of Objective Biomarkers**

   Currently, there are no definitive biomarkers or tests that can accurately measure the severity of PD. Diagnosis and assessment are primarily based on clinical observations and patient-reported symptoms. This subjective evaluation can lead to variations in determining the severity of the disease.

3. **Heterogeneity of Progression**

   PD is known for its heterogeneity in terms of the rate and pattern of disease progression. Some individuals may experience a slow progression of symptoms over many years, while others may have a more rapid decline. This heterogeneity makes it challenging to establish a standardized measurement of disease severity that applies universally.

4. **Patient Self-Reporting Bias**

   Patient self-reporting is often relied upon to evaluate the impact of symptoms and their severity. However, subjective reporting can be influenced by factors such as cognitive impairment, emotional well-being, and individual perception. This can introduce bias and inaccuracies in assessing the true severity of the disease.

5. **Interference from Medication**

   PD medications, such as L-dopa and dopamine agonists, can provide symptomatic relief and temporarily improve motor symptoms. However, these medications can also complicate the assessment of disease severity, as they can mask underlying symptoms and make it difficult to gauge the true extent of motor impairments.

Despite these challenges, healthcare professionals use various rating scales and assessments, such as the UPDRS and Hoehn and Yahr scale, to evaluate the severity of PD. These tools rely on a combination of clinical examination, patient interviews, and observation of motor and non-motor symptoms. Therefore, a clinical expression is only a photo in time, lacking complete information of before and after examination. Ongoing research as explained in [13], is focused on developing more objective measures, including the use of wearable sensors and advanced machine and deep techniques, to improve the accuracy of assessing PD and its severity.

References

1. Parkinson, J. An essay on the shaking palsy. *The Journal Of Neuropsychiatry And Clinical Neurosciences*. **14**, 223–236 (2002)
2. Ou, Z., Pan, J., Tang, S., Duan, D., Yu, D., Nong, H. & Wang, Z. Global trends in the incidence, prevalence, and years lived with disability of Parkinson's disease in 204 countries/territories from 1990 to 2019. *Frontiers In Public Health*. pp. 1994 (2021)
3. Parkinson's Change attitudes.Find a cure. Join us Parkinson's UK, Facts and figures about Parkinson's for journalists. (https://www.parkinsons.org.uk/about-us/media-and-pressoffice [Accessed September 4, 2023], 2020)
4. Okunoye, O., Kojima, G., Marston, L., Walters, K. & Schrag, A. Factors associated with hospitalisation among people with Parkinson's disease – A systematic review and meta-analysis. *Parkinsonism and Related Disorders*. **71** pp. 66–72 (2020)
5. Goetz, C., Tilley, B., Shaftman, S., Stebbins, G., Fahn, S., Martinez-Martin, P., Poewe, W., Sampaio, C., Stern, M., Dodel, R. & Others Movement Disorder Society-sponsored revision of the Unified Parkinson's Disease Rating Scale (MDS-UPDRS): scale presentation and clinimetric testing results. *Movement Disorders: Official Journal Of The Movement Disorder Society*. **23**, 2129–2170 (2008)
6. Yang, K., Xiong, W., Liu, F., Sun, Y., Luo, S., Ding, Z., Wu, J. & Wang, J. Objective and quantitative assessment of motor function in Parkinson's disease – from the perspective of practical applications. *Annals Of Translational Medicine*. **4** (2016)
7. Hallett, M. Parkinson's disease tremor: pathophysiology. *Parkinsonism & Related Disorders*. **18** pp. S85–S86 (2012)
8. Prochazka, A., Bennett, D., Stephens, M., Patrick, S., Sears-Duru, R., Roberts, T. & Jhamandas, J. Measurement of rigidity in Parkinson's disease. *Movement Disorders: Official Journal Of The Movement Disorder Society*. **12**, 24–32 (1997)
9. Barthel, C., Mallia, E., Debû, B., Bloem, B. & Ferraye, M. The practicalities of assessing freezing of gait. *Journal Of Parkinson's Disease*. **6**, 667–674 (2016)
10. Pozzi, N., Canessa, A., Palmisano, C., Brumberg, J., Steigerwald, F., Reich, M., Minafra, B., Pacchetti, C., Pezzoli, G., Volkmann, J. & Others Freezing of gait in Parkinson's disease reflects a sudden derangement of locomotor network dynamics. *Brain*. **142**, 2037–2050 (2019)
11. Allen, N., Schwarzel, A. & Canning, C. Recurrent falls in Parkinson's disease: a systematic review. *Parkinson's Disease*. **2013** (2013)
12. Thenganatt, M. & Louis, E. Distinguishing essential tremor from Parkinson's disease: bedside tests and laboratory evaluations. *Expert Review Of Neurotherapeutics*. **12**, 687–696 (2012)
13. Channa, A., Popescu, N. & Ciobanu, V. Wearable solutions for patients with Parkinson's disease and neurocognitive disorder: a systematic review. *Sensors*. **20**, 2713 (2020) **13**, 59–76 (2018)

Chapter 2
State-of-the-Art: Wearable Devices and Deep Learning Techniques for Parkinson's Disease

Abstract This chapter offers a comprehensive overview of the latest developments in wearable devices and Deep Learning (DL) techniques pertaining to the diagnosis and assessment of Parkinson's Disease (PD). It initiates by reviewing innovative wearable devices specifically designed to detect and monitor motor impairment in PD patients. These devices are pivotal for objective and continuous assessment, ensuring accurate and timely diagnosis. The chapter also highlights pertinent challenges in the field, encompassing remote monitoring limitations, the absence of cloud platforms, and constraints related to multiple nodes, impeding efficient data collection and analysis. In response to these challenges, a novel contribution is introduced in the form of an eHealth platform tailored for PD patients. The developed eHealth platform exemplifies the potential for advanced technologies to revolutionize the field and enhance the quality of life for individuals grappling with this debilitating neurological disorder.

2.1 Present Outlook and Evaluation of Parkinson's Disease

A standout among the most ceaseless and dynamic neurodegenerative diseases is PD. This is one of the most prevalent developmental issues of the focal sensory system, affecting approximately 3% of the global population over the age of 60 as by [1]. Certainly the most disabling symptom of the disease according to [2] is tremor. While RT is undoubtedly the most frequently examined type of tremor, investigating other types of tremors, such as PT or KT, is also extremely important. Approximately 80% of Parkinsonian patients have PT and KT tremors in addition to RT [3] and those tremors tend to worsen as they are getting older.

Medicines such as Carbidopa/Levodopa are used to reduce PD symptoms or arrest its progression, [4]. The treatments, however, show inherent limitations without knowledge of the disease's evolutionary state and produce side effects based on dosage and individual response of drug [5]. Hence it is necessary to know condition and severity of tremors in PD patients continuously. Tremor severity often indicates PD progress and severity. Treatment efficacy can also be evaluated using it. Currently, for the evaluation of symptoms' severity grade, the UPDRS [6] is commonly used

SpringerBriefs in Computer Science, https://doi.org/10.1007/978-3-031-45003-7_2

to diagnose PD, as well as to evaluate progress after the administration of new drugs and the modification of their dosages. In the UPDRS, the neurologist fills out a questionnaire based on his subjective observations and the patient's answers. According to the UPDRS, each activity or question is rated from 0 to 4, with 0 representing the absence of the disorder or no difficulty to perform a certain movement, and 4 representing the marked presence of the disorder or the marked difficulty to perform a particular movement. The summation of every item in the questionnaire results in a numerical evaluation of the disease. Because of the evaluation based on these rating scales, patients' disability diagnoses and classifications, including their tremor assessment, are still subject to error due to the varying personal interpretations and the lack of a universally applicable objective reference.

To eliminate the inherent subjectivity in physician evaluations and patient evaluations in UPDRS questionnaire filling, new techniques and systems need to be developed. Using these solutions, neurologists could generate objective reports and conduct repeatable tests on their patients. In this specialized medical field, effective tools must ensure ease of use for the medical practitioner and the patient, the non-invasiveness of measuring instruments, and the ability to produce reports in real-time or, at least, at times that are acceptable to the application. Additionally, such systems should provide home evaluations of the patient's symptoms as suggested by [7]. In this study, we developed, tested, and designed a prototype along with mobile cloud-based mHealth app, "A-WEAR", which has the capability of collecting quantitative and objective information about PD and enabling home-based assessment and monitoring of PD tremor severity.

2.2 Literature Review

The utilization of wearable devices for evaluating motor impairment, tracking disease advancement, and assessing DLAs in PD patients has garnered attention in research over the past decade. Numerous studies have explored the integration of wearable sensor devices and machine learning (ML) methods for various purposes. Despite these efforts, the successful implementation of technological systems in routine practice for aiding PD, online monitoring, and home-based observation remains an unattained goal.

As the disease of Parkinson's is still incurable. Yet there are some options available to give the patient some control over his/her motor and non-motor symptoms. PD can be treated non-invasively (using medicines) as well as invasively (using surgery). The medicines such as L-dopa used for PD treatments mainly hold back nerve impulses to control movements. A surgical or invasive method, such as Pallidotomy, Deep Brain Stimulation (DBS) [8], stimulates brain cells by placing electrical probes inside the brain.

Several works already exist on this approach, which introduced automated systems for PD severity estimation based on wearable sensor devices in conjunction with ML methods that perform better for objective assessment of PwPD. An example is [9] which proposed a method for tremor severity analysis by mounting a number of accelerometers on patients body and extracted features from the acquired signals and adopted Hidden Markov Model for prediction. This system was tested on 23 subjects and the obtained accuracy was 87% for quantifying tremor severity. But, in this system there is lack of tremor severity of level 4, which is an intensive one, thus the results are not generalised and can not assess all patients, along with that relatively low sensitivity and specificity i.e. 69% and 79% achieved for severity level 2. In [10], the authors proposed a wavelet-based approach for analysis of data from single wrist-worn smartwatches, and show high detection performance for tremor, bradykinesia, and dyskinesia using Support Vector Machine (SVM). However, features extracted aid to predict a total of three tremor severity levels i.e. 0, 1, 2 where level 2 represents tremor severities 2, 3 and 4. Table 2.1 depicts the state-of-the-art wearable devices proposed for monitoring of PD patients.

Since many attempts have been made to create wearable technology to assist in PD patient care, the majority of these solutions are still difficult to use in clinical settings in order to enhance PD diagnosis and management. Additionally, they are not suitable for usage by experts outside of the medical setting. The main difficulties stem from the fact that most wearables are battery-powered and must be charged; patients are concerned about small form factor devices that should be lighter in weight for better comfort; the devices still need improved security and privacy features; better communication capabilities; and, most importantly, quick real-time monitoring capacity. The problem of incorrect data distribution or a lack of density of a class or number of classes in the training model, which can result in false negative and misclassification, which is the main obstacle of using ML and DL algorithms in medical applications.

Given the primary focus of the researchers on short-term motor evaluation, the existing body of literature pertaining to PD assessment tools frequently contends with limited clinical data or encounters issues related to imbalanced datasets when validating conclusions.

To date, only one study, as documented by Polat et al. [20], has implemented an over-sampling technique for PD diagnosis through voice signal processing. Employing a Random Forest (RF) classifier alongside the over-sampling method, an accuracy of 94.89% was achieved. Notably, this study's scope did not encompass the classification of tremor severity. Similarly, Almahadin et al. [16] introduced an enhanced categorization methodology for tremor severity, integrating oversampling, under-sampling, and a hybrid configuration with artificial neural networks based on multi-layer perceptrons (ANN-MLP) and RF classifiers utilizing resampling approaches. Nonetheless, the implementation of ANN-MLP with Borderline SMOTE yielded a predictive accuracy of 93.81% for tremor prediction. This work primarily concentrated on preprocessing methodologies, employing resampling techniques in conjunction with machine learning, without offering a comprehensive end-to-end solution for remote monitoring of PD patients utilizing cloud computing and wearable devices.

Each proposed system either necessitated a substantial number of data collection nodes or was confined to system design aspects, often overlooking the continuous

Table 2.1 State-of-the-art of wearable devices per PD application area

Refs.	PD application scenario	Wearability	Mobile interface	Connectivity solutions	Online monitoring	Approach	Metrics
Dai et al. [11]	Bradykinesia and tremor assessment	Accelerometer, Gyroscope, Magnetometer	✗	✗	✗	SVM	Accuracy 0.97, Specificity 0.96, Sensitivity 1
Sigcha et al. [12]	RT assessment (severity 0, 1 and 2)	Triaxial accelerometers in smartwatch	✗	✗	✗	AdaBoost	Specificity 0.86, Sensitivity 0.86. AUC 0.93
Erb et al. [13]	Comparison of neurologists evaluation with results derived from wearable sensor data	Shimmer3	✗	✗	✗	Statistical methods (chi-squared test)	Compared with live video evaluation
Kim et al. [14]	Comparison of activity monitor from wrist and waist	ActiGraph GT3X+, ActiGraph, Penascola, FL	✗	✗	✗	Statistical analysis using in software (version 18: SPSS, Inc., Chicago, IL)	Wrist-worn activity monitor outperforms waist-worn counterpart
Hssayeni et al. [15]	Response of medication	Two KinetiSense sensors	✗	✗	✗	ON and OFF state pattern from sensor data	90.5% accuracy, 94.2% sensitivity, and 85.4% specificity
AlMahadin et al. [16]	Assessment of PD tremor across all severities	GENEActiv	✗	✗	✗	Resampling with ANN-MLP	Accuracy 0.95, Precision 0.95, Sensitivity 0.95, Specificity 0.98. F1-score 0.95, Gmean 0.96, IBA 0.93. AUC 0.99
Kim et al. [17]	Tremor assessment severities 0, 1, 2, (3, 4) together	Custom-developed device (SNUMAP) equipped with an accelerometer and gyroscope	✗	✗	✗	CNN model	Accuracy = 85%, Sensitivity = 79%, Precision 81%. Kappa coefficient = 85%. Correlation coefficient = 93%
Pan et al. [18]	Tremor and gait variability	Smartphone	✓	✓	✓	Decision support	The study emphasized system design but lacked details on cloud server data processing
Alhussein [19]	PD diagnosis and monitor health	Voice signals from mobile devices	✓	✓	✓	SVM	97.2% accuracy in detecting PD

online data processing and analysis of patients' motor systems. This limitation prevented the development of a holistic end-to-end solution for monitoring the motor activities of PD patients. An exhaustive review of pertinent literature reveals that this study stands as the inaugural endeavor to conceive a comprehensive ecosystem for PD patients, facilitating the continuous monitoring of their physical activities and the timely identification of PD severity.

In conclusion, despite the attempts to create wearable devices to assist in managing Parkinson's disease, most of these solutions have not yet found seamless integration into clinical practice for enhancing diagnosis and management. Additionally, they are not well-suited for use beyond hospital settings by professionals. Key challenges include the reliance on battery-powered devices that need frequent charging, limited battery life posing a constraint, patients' preference for compact and lightweight devices for comfort, the need for enhanced security and privacy features, improved communication capabilities, and crucially, real-time monitoring capability.

Implementing ML and DL algorithms in medical applications poses a significant challenge, especially in cases where data distribution is imbalanced or lacks class density, leading to misclassification and false negatives. Many prior studies related to PD assessment devices lack comprehensive clinical validation data, focusing primarily on short-term motor assessments using wearables in clinical environments. Another recurrent limitation in previous studies is the omission of various tremor levels that could aid in developing an objective measurement closer to clinical rating scales. Some studies only utilize task-specific data, excluding daily life activities, and pay little attention to wearable device efficiency or a robust cloud framework. Moreover, it is worth noting that the UPDRS assessment is time-consuming and demands specialized training, rendering it impractical for routine clinical practice. This contributes to inadequate PD management, resource wastage, and hindered routine clinical application.

2.3 Proposed Solution

To address these limitations, we have developed a bracelet capable of continuously recording various physical movements of a patient within a home environment. These movements encompass activities such as walking, turning, hand tremors at rest, and even actions like opening and closing a bottle cap. This data collection occurs over a 24 h period, with the device effectively and promptly storing the gathered information. Given the substantial volume of inertial sensor data collected from whole-day home monitoring, which can be overwhelming for a single computer to handle, we have devised a solution to efficiently manage data storage and rapid computation. This involves the creation of a cloud computing environment, specifically designed to store and analyze the extensive dataset swiftly using a specialized deep learning algorithm. The outcomes of this computation are transferred to end-users upon request, ensuring utmost security in the process.

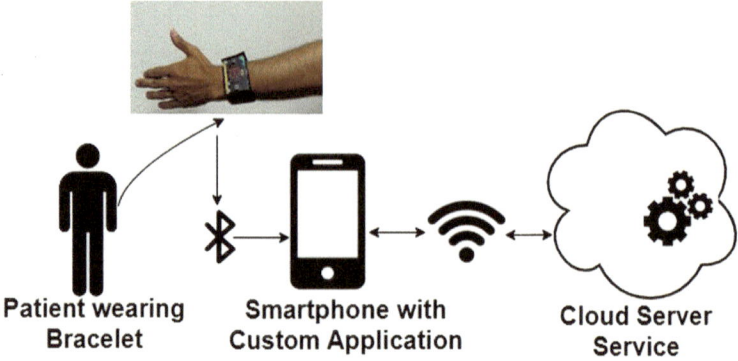

Fig. 2.1 The block diagram of the proposed PD monitoring system

In this research endeavor, we present a compact and energy-efficient smart bracelet device. This device seamlessly interfaces with smartphones using Wi-Fi or Bluetooth Low Energy (BLE), while consistently uploading data to a cloud platform. Within the cloud environment, the gathered data undergoes computational analysis, with a focus on segregating PD patient data based on severity levels for optimized management of L-dopa dosage. The proposed framework, depicted in Fig. 2.1, prioritizes user privacy and data security. All data exchanges between the ServiceNow platform (a cloud-based IT service management platform [21]) are encrypted, and access occurs exclusively through predefined Azure Sphere APIs (Application Programming Interfaces).

To recap, this innovative solution contributes in the following ways:

- A comprehensive system designed for the continuous monitoring and analysis of PD symptoms, offering full autonomy and the ability to track motions in everyday life.
- A structured framework for evaluating the severity of tremor and bradykinesia symptoms using a wearable bracelet equipped with wireless inertial sensors and cloud connectivity. This framework enables remote monitoring by medical professionals, facilitating remote patient management.
- The objective of this study revolves around the development of a DL model capable of predicting the response of PD patients to L-dopa medication. The insights garnered from this analysis aim to enhance the patients' QoL by providing valuable information to their clinicians for optimizing medication dosages, thereby mitigating the potential risks associated with medication side effects.

References

1. N. Ball, W.-P. Teo, S. Chandra, and J. Chapman, *Parkinson's disease and the environment*, *Frontiers in neurology*, pp. 218, 2019.
2. P. Pierleoni, A. Belli, O. Bazgir, L. Maurizi, M. Paniccia, and L. Palma, "A smart inertial system for 24h monitoring and classification of tremor and freezing of gait in Parkinson's disease," *IEEE Sensors Journal*, vol. 19, no. 23, pp. 11612–11623, 2019, publisher: IEEE.
3. L.J. Findley, M.A. Gresty, and G.M. Halmagyi, *Tremor, the cogwheel phenomenon and clonus in Parkinson's disease.*, *Journal of Neurology, Neurosurgery & Psychiatry*, vol. 44, no. 6, pp. 534–546, 1981.
4. M. Senek, S.-M. Aquilonius, H. Askmark, F. Bergquist, R. Constantinescu, A. Ericsson, S. Lycke, A. Medvedev, M. Memedi, F. Ohlsson, and others, *Levodopa/carbidopa microtablets in Parkinson's disease: a study of pharmacokinetics and blinded motor assessment*, *European journal of clinical pharmacology*, vol. 73, no. 5, pp. 563–571, 2017.
5. R. Dhall and D.L. Kreitzman, *Advances in levodopa therapy for Parkinson disease: review of RYTARY (carbidopa and levodopa) clinical efficacy and safety*, *Neurology*, vol. 86, no. 14 Supplement 1, pp. S13–S24, 2016.
6. Movement Disorder Society Task Force on Rating Scales for Parkinson's Disease, *The unified Parkinson's disease rating scale (UPDRS): status and recommendations*, *Movement Disorders*, vol. 18, no. 7, pp. 738–750, 2003.
7. A. Almogren, *An automated and intelligent Parkinson disease monitoring system using wearable computing and cloud technology*, *Cluster Computing*, vol. 22, no. 1, pp. 2309–2316, 2019.
8. M. L. Kringelbach, N. Jenkinson, S. L. F. Owen, and T. Z. Aziz, "Translational principles of deep brain stimulation," *Nature Reviews Neuroscience*, vol. 8, no. 8, pp. 623–635, 2007.
9. G. Rigas, A. Tzallas, M. G. Tsipouras, P. Bougia, E. E. Tripoliti, D. Baga, D. I. Fotiadis, S. G. Tsouli, and S. Konitsiotis, "Assessment of tremor activity in the Parkinson's disease using a set of wearable sensors," *IEEE Transactions on Information Technology in Biomedicine*, vol. 16, no. 3, pp. 478–487, 2012.
10. A. Wagner, N. Fixler, and Y. S. Resheff, "A wavelet-based approach to monitoring Parkinson's disease symptoms," in *2017 IEEE International Conference on Acoustics, Speech and Signal Processing (ICASSP)*, pp. 5980–5984, 2017.
11. H. Dai, G. Cai, Z. Lin, Z. Wang, and Q. Ye, "Validation of inertial sensing-based wearable device for tremor and bradykinesia quantification," *IEEE Journal of Biomedical and Health Informatics*, vol. 25, no. 4, pp. 997–1005, 2020.
12. L. Sigcha, I. Pavón, N. Costa, S. Costa, M. Gago, P. Arezes, J. M. López, and G. De Arcas, "Automatic resting tremor assessment in Parkinson's disease using smartwatches and multitask convolutional neural networks," *Sensors*, vol. 21, no. 1, pp. 291, 2021.
13. M. K. Erb, D. R. Karlin, B. K. Ho, K. C. Thomas, F. Parisi, G. P. Vergara-Diaz, J.-F. Daneault, P. W. Wacnik, H. Zhang, T. Kangarloo, and others, "mHealth and wearable technology should replace motor diaries to track motor fluctuations in Parkinson's disease," *NPJ digital medicine*, vol. 3, no. 1, pp. 1–10, 2020.
14. D. W. Kim, L. M. Hassett, V. Nguy, and N. E. Allen, "A Comparison of Activity Monitor Data from Devices Worn on the Wrist and the Waist in People with Parkinson's Disease," *Movement disorders clinical practice*, vol. 6, no. 8, pp. 693–699, 2019.
15. M. D. Hssayeni, M. A. Burack, and J. Jimenez-Shahed, "Assessment of response to medication in individuals with Parkinson's disease," *Medical engineering & physics*, vol. 67, pp. 33–43, 2019.
16. G. AlMahadin, A. Lotfi, M. M. Carthy, and P. Breedon, "Enhanced Parkinson's disease tremor severity classification by combining signal processing with resampling techniques," *SN Computer Science*, vol. 3, no. 1, pp. 1–21, 2022.
17. H. B. Kim, W. W. Lee, A. Kim, H. J. Lee, H. Y. Park, H. S. Jeon, S. K. Kim, B. Jeon, and K. S. Park, "Wrist sensor-based tremor severity quantification in Parkinson's disease using

convolutional neural network," *Computers in biology and medicine*, vol. 95, pp. 140–146, 2018.

18. D. Pan, R. Dhall, A. Lieberman, and D. B. Petitti, "A mobile cloud-based Parkinson's disease assessment system for home-based monitoring," *JMIR mHealth and uHealth*, vol. 3, no. 1, pp. e3956, 2015.

19. M. Alhussein, "Monitoring Parkinson's disease in smart cities," *IEEE Access*, vol. 5, pp. 19835–19841, 2017.

20. K. Polat, "A hybrid approach to Parkinson disease classification using speech signal: the combination of smote and random forests," in *2019 Scientific Meeting on Electrical-Electronics & Biomedical Engineering and Computer Science (EBBT)*, pp. 1–3, 2019.

21. Lawton, G. Developing software online with platform-as-a-service technology. *Computer.* **41**, 13–15 (2008)

Chapter 3
Design and Engineering of a Medical Wearable Device for Parkinson's Disease Management

Abstract The emergence of Internet of Things (IoT)-based wearable devices has ushered in new possibilities for the detection, diagnosis, and quantification of Parkinson's Disease (PD). These devices predominantly rely on inertial sensors and computational algorithms, offering promising advancements. However, they also introduce fresh challenges, including concerns related to security, privacy, connectivity, and power efficiency. From a clinical perspective, effective monitoring of patients' motor function is crucial for adjusting L-dopa doses, avoiding adverse effects, and mitigating motor activity deterioration. Adapting to variations in motor functions observed between different appointments poses a significant hurdle for clinicians, potentially leading to incorrect decisions. The principal objective of this chapter is to establish a comprehensive ecosystem that streamlines enhanced evaluation of PD stages and disease progression, especially concerning tremor and bradykinesia. This chapter endeavors to craft a holistic ecosystem capable of capturing motion data associated with PD and securely transmitting it to the cloud for storage, data processing, and severity estimation, all facilitated by specially developed learning algorithms.

3.1 Differentiating Factors: Designing a Custom Bracelet for Parkinson's Disease Patients Amidst Existing Wearable Devices

In recent times, there has been an upsurge in the availability of fitness wearable devices incorporating Inertial Measurement Units (IMUs), exemplified by products such as the Apple Watch (Apple Inc., Cupertino, San Francisco, CA, USA), Samsung Gear S (Samsung, Seoul, Korea), Mio Alpha (MioLabs Inc., Santa Clara, CA, USA), among others. These devices offer the capability to monitor a range of health metrics including daily step count, oxygen saturation (SpO_2), skin temperature, breathing rate, resting heart rate, sleep activity, and heart rate variability. As highlighted by Auepanwiriyakul et al. [9], these consumer-grade wearables equipped with motion-tracking capabilities are convenient for capturing the natural behaviors of clinical

A. Channa and N. Popescu, *Deep Learning in Smart eHealth Systems*, SpringerBriefs in Computer Science, https://doi.org/10.1007/978-3-031-45003-7_3

Table 3.1 Available wrist worn wearable devices for PD patients

Refs.	Device	Continuous monitoring	Unsupervised method	Online monitoring	Home monitoring	Application scenario
López-Blanco et al. [1]	Smartwatch3 (SW3) sony	✘	✘	✘	✘	Quantification of RT using wrist sensors
Heijmans et al. [2]	MOX5 wearables (Maastricht Instruments, Maastricht, The Netherlands)	✓	✓	✘	✓	Tremor detection using wrist sensors in DLAs
Hssayeni et al. [3]	One motion sensor (Great Lakes NeuroTechnologies Inc., Cleveland, OH, USA)	✓	✘	✘	✓	Investigated tremor severity in free body movements
Hssayeni et al. [4]	Two KinetiSense motion sensors	✓	✓	✘	✘	Response of medication over symptoms severity
San-Segundo et al. [5]	Wrist-worn wearable accelerometer	✓	✓	✘	✓	Assessment of disease progression and treatment effects
Kim et al. [6]	ActiGraph GT3X+, ActiGraph, Penascola, FL	✓	✓	✘	✓	Comparison of activity monitor from wrist and waist
Erb et al. [7]	Shimmer3	✓	✓	✘	✓	Estimates the motor state derived from wearable sensor data, participants' self-report of their motor state, and the timing of L-dopa
Zwartjes et al. [8]	MT9 inertial sensors (3-D accelerometers and 3-D gyroscopes, Xsens Technologies BV, Enschede, The Netherlands)	✓	✓	✘	✓	Monitoring of motor activities ans symptoms

patients. However, a pertinent question arises: are these wearable devices equally suitable for assessing the condition of Parkinson's Disease (PD) patients?

It is notable that these smart wearable devices possess the capacity to accurately count steps and ascertain stride lengths, making them well-suited for fitness tracking and managing the daily routines of individuals. However, the unique variability exhibited by PD patients distinguishes them from the general patient population. Consequently, while these commercial smart wearables can provide valuable feedback concerning activity levels, they fall short in offering an objective assessment tailored to the specific needs of PD patients. Instead, their potential is predominantly harnessed in aiding rehabilitation efforts.

In this chapter, we delve into the compatibility of contemporary fitness wearables with PD patient assessment, exploring their capabilities, limitations, and the prospects they hold within the realm of Parkinson's Disease management. Through an in-depth examination, we aim to elucidate the role of these devices in contributing to the holistic understanding of PD patient health and well-being.

Alternative commercially available prototypes, including Fitbit, Garmin, Actigraph, and Xsens, present enhanced patient comfort within a home setting. These prototypes are employed by subjects without the need for extensive evaluation, boasting extended battery life and serving as protracted activity monitoring systems for Parkinson's Disease (PD) patients. In a study by Wendel et al. [10], a cross-sectional assessment of the accuracy of consumer-grade activity trackers (Fitbit Zip, Fitbit Surge, Jawbone Up 2, and Jawbone Up Move) was conducted on individuals with PD during simulated ambulation tasks, revealing the Fitbit Zip as the most accurate device across all tasks, while the Jawbone Up Move exhibited the lowest accuracy.

Similarly, Lamont et al. [11] juxtaposed the results of Fitbit Charge HR and Garmin Vivosmart HR with ActivPAL3, determining Garmin to have a lower error rate than Fitbit. However, the assortment of prototypes and systems highlighted in Table 3.1 collectively lacks a dedicated cloud-based evaluation environment. Consequently, a demand persists for a comprehensive system that not only quantifies illness severity but also facilitates the rehabilitation of People with Parkinson's Disease (PwPD) within an uncontrolled environment. This system should allow patients to employ it autonomously during both ON and OFF stages without supervision.

Additional wrist-worn wearable solutions for PD patients are documented in Table 3.1. It is apparent that each solution carries specific limitations, often presenting affordability challenges. In contrast, our proposed device is reasonably priced at around 400 euros, offering a cost-effective yet robust solution due to the innovative architecture underpinning its design.

3.2 First Iteration: Design and Functionality of the Initial A-WEAR Bracelet

3.3 Description of Measurement System

In this research, we employed a hand bracelet as the fundamental measurement tool. This bracelet serves to gather data pertaining to the hand movements exhibited by both PD patients and individuals without the condition. The design of the bracelet revolves around a compact microcontroller, which efficiently records real-time information from a specialized sensor module encompassing an accelerometer and a gyroscope. The captured output values are subsequently stored onto a micro SD card. The schematic representation of the A-WEAR bracelet's block design is illustrated in Fig. 3.1.

The elements employed in constructing this bracelet encompass:

1. The Cmod MX1 microcontroller, featuring a microchip PIC32MX150F128D microprocessor.
2. The Pmod NAV module, housing a 3-axis accelerometer and 3-axis gyroscope sensor.
3. The Pmod micro SD module, designated for data storage on the micro SD card.

Figure 3.2 depicts the components employed in the bracelet's development. In this setup, the Pmod NAV facilitates the acquisition of a range of orientation-related data, providing users with the ability to accurately determine the module's precise position and orientation. This module supplies raw data, which, in conjunction with the processing speed enabled by the 40 MHz PIC microprocessor, allows for the calculation of acceleration (G) and degrees per second (dps) values from the accelerometer and gyroscope. These calculated values are subsequently stored on the micro SD card. This approach ensures that the neural and machine learning (ML) classifiers can directly operate with readable data, thus avoiding the need to expend time on converting raw data. Both the Pmod NAV and the micro SD module utilize the SPI (serial peripheral interface) protocol to communicate with the microcontroller.

The microcontroller captures real-time data over a fixed time span, sufficient to achieve an accurate data interpretation. For the initial version of the device, two status LEDs were incorporated. One LED serves as an indicator that the bracelet

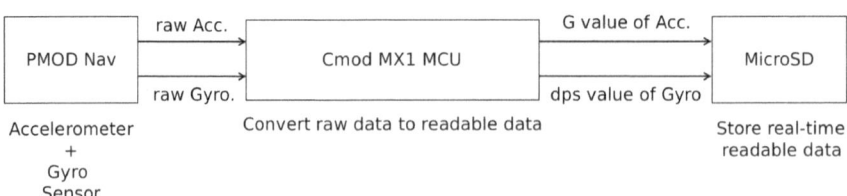

Fig. 3.1 Bracelet's block design

Fig. 3.2 Constituents
employed in crafting the
A-WEAR bracelet

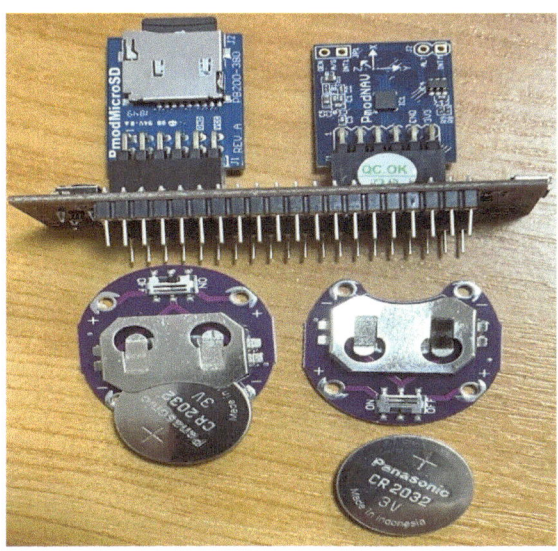

Fig. 3.2 Constituents employed in crafting the A-WEAR bracelet

has been calibrated and all modules are functioning correctly. Once the first LED is illuminated, it signifies the initiation of data acquisition. Subsequently, when the second LED lights up, it indicates the completion of data acquisition, allowing the micro SD card to be safely removed for subsequent data analysis. The design of the bracelet has been carefully crafted to ensure ease of wear on the wrist for patients. To power the device, two 3V batteries, commonly found in digital watches, were utilized, providing a battery life of approximately 3 hours. It's important to note that this bracelet is solely intended for data collection purposes. Preliminary developmental stages of the bracelet are presented in Fig. 3.3a, while the final prototype is displayed in Fig. 3.3b.

3.4 Enhanced Functionality: Upgraded Features of the Advanced Parkinson's Disease Bracelet

For objective assessment of Prakinsonian motor symptoms, the preliminary version of bracelet [12] acquires data of the hand movements of the patients. The bracelet is developed using a small form-factor microcontroller that reads real-time data from a special sensor module that contains an accelerometer and a gyroscope and transfer the data to SD card. This device helps in collecting data from individuals and getting diagnosis of PD. The device was tested on a group of patients with PD (PwPD). All the participants performed specific motor tasks while wearing this bracelet for few minutes.

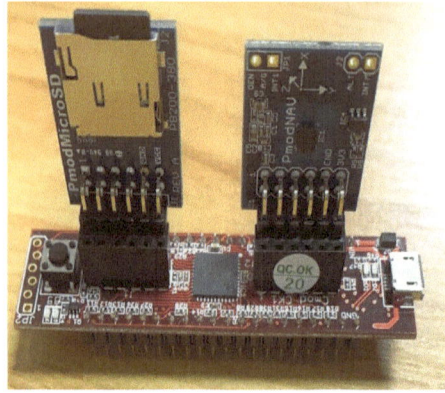 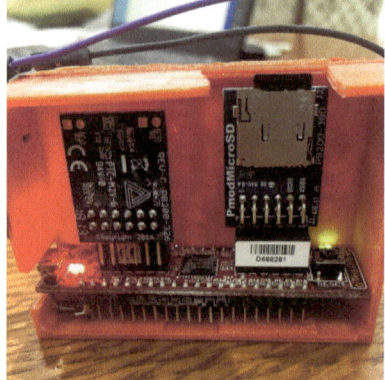

(a) Preliminary stage   (b) Final prototype

Fig. 3.3 A-WEAR bracelet developmental stages

Fig. 3.4 The latest version
of A-WEAR bracelet

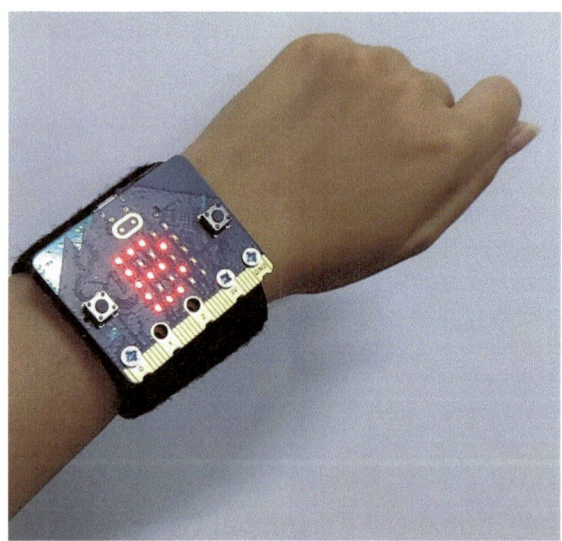

The drawbacks in previous version of A-WEAR bracelet are: it just helps in collection of motor signals for few minutes, has dimension 33 mm × 22 mm × 2.5 mm. The operating voltage requirement is 3 V. Considering these features and to provide more feasibility to patients and doctors, our latest version of the A-WEAR bracelet as shown in Fig. 3.4 is developed using BBC micro:bit which is a development board that uses a microcontroller. The Micro:bit V2 is a small, easy-to-use ARM Cortex M4. It is equipped with 25 LEDs, on which messages or images can be displayed, with an accelerometer to detect movements, a compass, Bluetooth, and two buttons that can be used to interact with the user. The dimensions of bracelet is half of credit

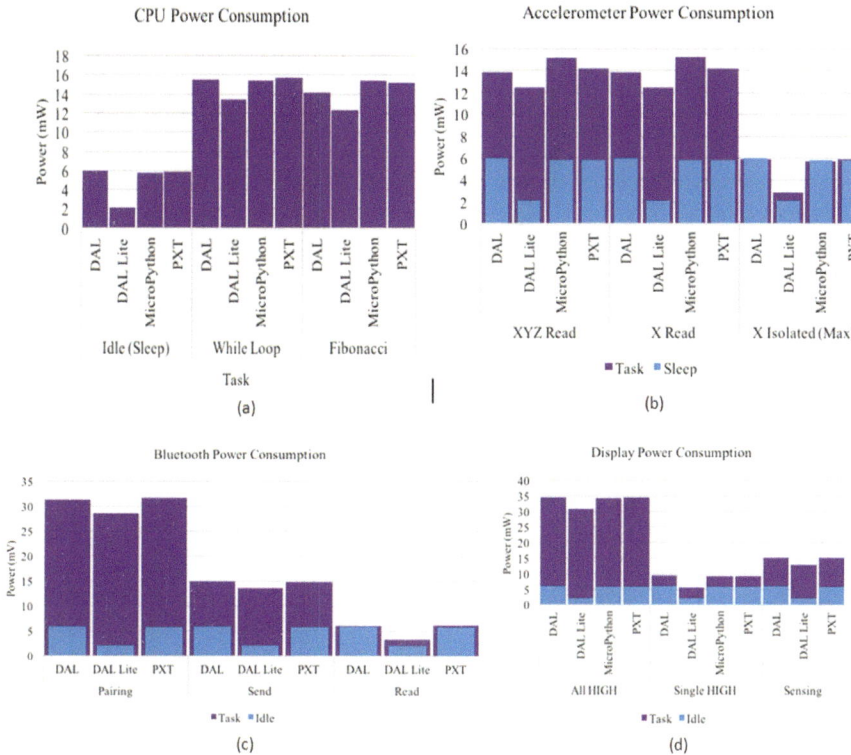

Fig. 3.5 Power consumption of CPU, BLE, matrix lex and accelerometer

card size and requires just 1.8 V to operate. The bracelet connects to android phone using BLE and updates the results continuously on A-WEAR mobile application.

The patient wears it on his most effected limb, and turns ON the bracelet using the slide button. There are two push buttons A and B (are programmable). When both are pressed the bracelet restart. First bracelet needed to be connected with smart phone with our A-WEAR mobile app using Bluetooth (BLE). when the bracelet connects with the smart phone the sign of **C** appears on display which is 5 × 5 array of LEDs and programmed to give the message of **B** as Bluetooth, **C** as connected, **D** as Disconnected and √ as data is successfully collected and so on. The micro:bit microcontroller was used as an upgrade that assures its low power consumption, small form factor which suits perfectly the wearable design, and out of the box needed peripherals like accelerometer, BLE, Matrix display. The operating voltage range of the micro:bit device as a whole is between 1.7 V min and 3.6 V max. The on-board current budget will vary depending on the use of the display, the Bluetooth, microphone, speaker and other peripherals. As detailed by the vendor, it should allow a worst case budget of 30 mA for when all on-board peripherals are in use (which is not the case for this application).

The point of interest elements of the controller that are used are the CPU, BLE, Matrix Lex and accelerometer which have the following power consumption as shown in Fig. 3.5. The worst case scenario of maximum usage of all the above elements would result in about a total of 97 mW of power consumption. As we use as power supply a CR2032 battery with a voltage of 3 V and a capacity of up to 240 mAh, the estimated battery life at maximum usage on the microcontroller and its peripherals would result in about 5–6 hrs of usage. Of course this would be the worst case scenario where the microcontroller would be used continuously with the highest power consumption tasks.

From our experiments with normal usage, meaning that several readings are performed per day (10–20 readings of 1 min each), the battery lasted more than two weeks before it needed to be changed. The micro:bit V2 uses Bluetooth 5.0 stack with Bluetooth Low Energy (BLE). Like other Bluetooth devices, it runs on the ISM (Industrial Scientific Medical) band. It operates between 2.4 and 2.41 GHz. The frequency range is divided into 50×2 MHz bands by BLE, of which 40 are utilized. These have the numbers 0–39 and are known as channels. The usage of channels 37, 38, and 39 is known as "advertising." When linked, devices utilise the additional channels in a certain order that is managed by a function called adaptive frequency hopping. This aids in lessening the effects of radio user congestion. Data transfer rates will only be a few hundred Kilobytes per second at best, which is enough as every accelerometer read defined at the sample rate, the X, Y, Z data is sent to the A-WEAR mobile application to be added in the final csv file.

After the defined reading period completes, the A-WEAR app takes all the received accelerometer readings and saves them in a CSV file which is then uploaded to ServiceNow in a separate record for each reading session. A reading session recorded for 1 min for example produces a file of about 90 KB, and the necessary upload time of the file via REST API to the ServiceNow platform takes under a second.

After connection, the mobile app allow entering the patient ID, name and other important details i.e. sampling frequency or time period for data transfer and then 'Start' can be chosen. After starting it, the data that is collected can be downloaded on the phone and also can be uploaded to the cloud platform where the CSV files go into the training and analysis phase and the PD tremors severity is estimated. This is the procedure of the proposed and developed end-to-end system to track the PD tremor symptom that is fully autonomous and capable of continuously monitoring and analyzing motions during everyday life.

References

1. López-Blanco, R., Velasco, M., Méndez-Guerrero, A., Romero, J., Del Castillo, M., Serrano, J., Rocon, E. & Benito-León, J. Smartwatch for the analysis of rest tremor in patients with Parkinson's disease. *Journal Of The Neurological Sciences.* **401** pp. 37–42 (2019)

2. Heijmans, M., Habets, J., Kuijf, M., Kubben, P. & Herff, C. Evaluation of Parkinson's Disease at Home: Predicting Tremor from Wearable Sensors. *2019 41st Annual International Conference Of The IEEE Engineering In Medicine And Biology Society (EMBC)*. pp. 584–587 (2019)
3. Hssayeni, M., Jimenez-Shahed, J., Burack, M. & Ghoraani, B. Wearable sensors for estimation of parkinsonian tremor severity during free body movements. *Sensors*. **19**, 4215 (2019)
4. Hssayeni, M., Burack, M., Jimenez-Shahed, J. & Ghoraani, B. Assessment of response to medication in individuals with Parkinson's disease. *Medical Engineering & Physics*. **67** pp. 33–43 (2019)
5. San-Segundo, R., Zhang, A., Cebulla, A., Panev, S., Tabor, G., Stebbins, K., Massa, R., Whitford, A., Torre, F. & Hodgins, J. Parkinson's Disease Tremor Detection in the Wild Using Wearable Accelerometers. *Sensors*. **20**, 5817 (2020)
6. Kim, D., Hassett, L., Nguy, V. & Allen, N. A Comparison of Activity Monitor Data from Devices Worn on the Wrist and the Waist in People with Parkinson's Disease. *Movement Disorders Clinical Practice*. **6**, 693–699 (2019)
7. Erb, M., Karlin, D., Ho, B., Thomas, K., Parisi, F., Vergara-Diaz, G., Daneault, J., Wacnik, P., Zhang, H., Kangarloo, T. & Others mHealth and wearable technology should replace motor diaries to track motor fluctuations in Parkinson's disease. *NPJ Digital Medicine*. **3**, 1–10 (2020)
8. Zwartjes, D., Heida, T., Van Vugt, J., Geelen, J. & Veltink, P. Ambulatory monitoring of activities and motor symptoms in Parkinson's disease. *IEEE Transactions On Biomedical Engineering*. **57**, 2778–2786 (2010)
9. Auepanwiriyakul, C., Waibel, S., Songa, J., Bentley, P. & Faisal, A. Accuracy and Acceptability of Wearable Motion Tracking for Inpatient Monitoring Using Smartwatches. *Sensors*. **20**, 7313 (2020)
10. Wendel, N., Macpherson, C., Webber, K., Hendron, K., DeAngelis, T., Colon-Semenza, C. & Ellis, T. Accuracy of activity trackers in Parkinson disease: should we prescribe them?. *Physical Therapy*. **98**, 705–714 (2018)
11. Lamont, R., Daniel, H., Payne, C. & Brauer, S. Accuracy of wearable physical activity trackers in people with Parkinson's disease. *Gait & Posture*. **63** pp. 104–108 (2018)
12. Channa, A., Ifrim, R., Popescu, D. & Popescu, N. A-WEAR bracelet for detection of hand tremor and bradykinesia in Parkinson's patients. *Sensors*. **21**, 981 (2021)

Chapter 4
Deep Learning Models for Parkinson's Disease Severity Evaluation

Abstract This chapter conducts a comprehensive exploration into the application of Machine Learning (ML) and Deep Learning (DL) algorithms for the diagnosis and assessment of Parkinson's Disease (PD) severity through remote and continuous monitoring. The chapter is divided into two sections, outlining the methodology and results of the study. In the first section, an A-WEAR bracelet is employed for the objective assessment of tremor and bradykinesia in PD subjects and healthy older adults. To distinguish patients from healthy controls, temporal and spectral features are extracted, with non-linear temporal and spectral features demonstrating substantial differences. Both supervised and unsupervised ML classifiers yield favorable results. In the second section, a resampling technique is adopted to address the issue of an unbalanced dataset. Time and frequency-based features are extracted, and the signals are analyzed using the CatBoost classifier. This approach yields an impressive accuracy rate of 96%. The findings of this study substantially contribute to the development of a reliable and accurate framework for assessing PD severity.

4.1 Identifying Hand Tremor and Bradykinesia with Machine Learning and A-WEAR Bracelet

4.2 Overview

In this research work, we employed a comprehensive methodology where we extracted time and frequency based features and employed supervised and unsupervised ML classifier for the automatic diagnosis of PD. In contrast, our alternative approach involved utilizing time-frequency signals adopting resampling methods and adopting Catboost classifier for remote continuous assessment of motors symptoms. By comparing both approaches, we were able to discern the strengths and limitations of each method, shedding light on their respective effectiveness in our study.

A. Channa and N. Popescu, *Deep Learning in Smart eHealth Systems*,
SpringerBriefs in Computer Science, https://doi.org/10.1007/978-3-031-45003-7_4

4.2.1 The Subjects and the Acquisition Procedure

A total of 40 participants took part in this study, comprising 20 individuals diagnosed with PD exhibiting varying degrees of tremor and bradykinesia severity, while the remaining participants constituted age-matched healthy controls. The group of PD patients included 5 males and 15 females who were invited to participate. Their relevant details are as follows: mean age ± standard deviation (SD): 71.65 ± 6.872 years old; average MDS/UPDRS scores ± SD: 18.91 ± 7.831; average Hoehn and Yahr (H&Y) stage ± SD: 1.65 ± 0.526, and disease duration in years ± SD: 7.7 ± 4.495. On the other hand, the group of healthy participants consisted of 16 males and 4 females, with a mean age ± SD of 70.25 ± 6.307 years old. Among the 20 patients, 10 exhibited only the tremor symptom without bradykinesia signs, while the remaining 10 showed bradykinesia symptoms without tremor during the performance of activities as outlined in [1]. Table 4.1 presents the most relevant demographic and clinical information of the subjects. The data acquisition process comprised two separate sessions. In the first session, activities conducive to tremor detection were undertaken, while the second session involved activities aimed at bradykinesia detection. Due to Covid-19 precautions, the data acquisition was conducted in a home environment under the supervision of a neurologist. All participants in the study provided informed consent and were instructed to perform the tasks accurately. The bracelet was attached to the predominantly affected hand of the PD patients.

Part 1: Validation of Tremor Detection

RT is one of the most pronounced tremors observed in individuals with PD, with around 25% of PD patients also experiencing action and postural tremors. The severity of tremors tends to increase when all these types are present in a PD patient. The assessment of different types of tremors involves specific testing procedures:

1. To assess RT in its upper limits, patients are instructed to rest their forearms comfortably on their thighs for one minute. RT often manifests as a rhythmic flexion-extension movement of the wrist/hand, a back-and-forth rotation of the forearm, or a continuous rolling motion of the thumb and index finger.
2. Postural tremor arises when a patient maintains a position against the force of gravity, typically exhibiting a frequency range between 4 and 12 Hz [2]. For testing PT, the patient is initially asked to fully extend the elbow and then flex the arm forward to a 90° angle. Subsequently, the participant is instructed to spread their fingers as wide as possible and maintain this posture for a minute. This particular duration is important, as postural tremors in PD tend to emerge within a minute of assuming the position.
3. Action or kinetic tremor manifests only during the execution of a specific activity. The frequency of KT generally falls within the range of 2–7 Hz [3]. The finger-to-nose test is commonly employed to assess action tremor. During this task, patients are guided to alternately touch their nose and an extended finger. It's important for

Table 4.1 Demographic and clinical details of healthy control and patient with Parkinson disease

Healthy control age (Gender)	Patient with PD			
	Age (Gender)	UPDRS (0–56)	H & Y (1–5)	Disease duration (Years)
75 (F)	62 (F)	23	1.5	7
64 (M)	66 (F)	5	1.5	6
75 (M)	72 (F)	9	2	6
80 (F)	73 (F)	26	2	20
83 (M)	78 (M)	5	1	13
65 (M)	65 (M)	27	1	14
65 (M)	79 (F)	23	1	5
61 (M)	69 (F)	15	2	3
63 (M)	80 (M)	25	2	8
70 (M)	81 (M)	18	1.5	4
70 (F)	60 (F)	20	2	11
76 (M)	80 (F)	26	2	10
67 (M)	65 (F)	7	1	1
66 (F)	75 (M)	30	1	2
62 (M)	72 (F)	18	1	7
66 (M)	63 (F)	22	1.5	3
74 (M)	66 (F)	15	1.5	9
71 (M)	83 (F)	15	2.5	10
72 (M)	75 (F)	32	2.5	5
80 (M)	69 (F)	30	2.5	10
70.25 (±6.307)	71.65 (±6.872)	18.91 (±7.831)	1.65 (±0.526)	7.7 (±4.495)

patients to fully extend their arm and avoid quick movements, as this maximizes the likelihood of triggering the tremor. The test is performed for a duration of 60 seconds for each participant.

Part 2: Validation of Bradykinesia Detection

Bradykinesia stands as another cardinal motor symptom prevalent among PD patients. To assess its presence, specific exercises are employed by the patients:

1. Finger Tapping: A primary evaluation involves finger tapping, where the participant, whether a control subject or a PD patient, is seated and instructed to repeatedly tap their thumb against their index finger as rapidly and frequently as possible for a duration of 60 s.

2. Fist Open and Close: For the assessment of bradykinesia, the participant maintains their arms in the same position as during the hand movement test. However, this time, the patient is prompted to alternately open and close their hand as swiftly and extensively as they can. This activity is performed with the largest range of motion achievable and is carried out for a duration of one minute.
3. Pronation/Supination: Bradykinesia is also evaluated for each upper extremity using the pronation/supination test. In this test, the seated patient raises their elbow to chest level, flexes it to a 90° angle with the palm facing upward, and then proceeds to move the hand and forearm as quickly as possible, covering the widest possible range of motion. This movement pattern is sustained for a duration of 60 s. Similar to finger tapping, this evaluation is conducted for both sides of the body.

4.3   Methodology

Following the acquisition procedure, a total of 40 recordings were gathered, comprising 20 recordings from healthy subjects and an equal split of 10 recordings each from patients exhibiting tremor and those manifesting bradykinesia symptoms. The initial step involved processing the collected data through a filtering procedure designed to eliminate drift, outliers, and unwanted frequencies. This filtration process was guided by previous research, which delineated the frequency bands associated with tremor.

Subsequently, the data underwent visualization to accentuate the distinctions between the data from healthy participants and subjects grappling with tremor and bradykinesia symptoms in their daily lives. Once the visualization was accomplished, the focus shifted to feature extraction. The extracted features were then subjected to machine learning (ML) classifiers, which performed the task of classifying and detecting tremor and bradykinesia. An overarching schematic representation of the entire process is presented in Fig. 4.1, outlining the sequence of steps involved.

4.3.1   Data Analysis

Signal Processing

The recorded signal has a sampling rate of 100 Hz, which accommodates the fact that the tremor frequency of upper extremities typically remains below 13 Hz. Accordingly, as indicated by [4], the chosen 100 Hz sampling frequency is deemed adequate for capturing PD-related motor features. Before proceeding with visualization and feature extraction, a preliminary step involves filtering all the recorded signals using a Butterworth bandpass Infinite Impulse Response (IIR) filter of 10 order. The cut-off frequencies for this filter are set at 2 and 20 Hz.

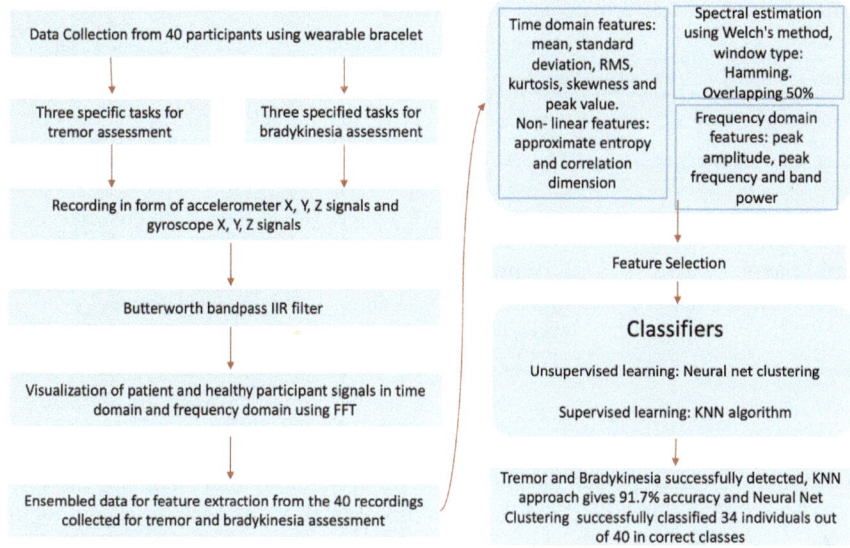

Fig. 4.1 Illustration of the whole process for detection of tremor and bradykinesia

Signal Visualization

To comprehensively analyze the signal, visualization becomes an essential step to discern the key distinctions between signals from healthy participants and those with PD. This process aids in the elimination of undesirable noise and frequencies, facilitates the design of precise filters, and enhances the understanding of signal behavior across both the time and frequency domains.

4.3.2 Feature Extraction and Importance

To ensure precise outcomes, the presence of appropriate features that effectively characterize tremor and bradykinesia is crucial. As illustrated in Fig. 4.4, we meticulously processed the gathered data and organized it cohesively, enabling the extraction of both temporal and spectral features.

Time domain features

Time domain features are divided into two parts i.e linear and non-linear features. The linear features which we extracted are: mean, standard deviation, root mean square (RMS), kurtosis, skewness and peak value while the non-linear features are

Table 4.2 Mathematical representation of the features

Features	Mahematical representation	Commands
Mean	$\mu = \frac{1}{N} \sum_{i=1}^{N} x_i$	Mean
Standard deviation	$\sigma = \sqrt{\frac{1}{N-1} \sum_{i=1}^{N} |x_i - \mu|}$	Std
Root mean square (RMS)	$X_{rms} = \sqrt{\frac{1}{N} \sum_{i=1}^{N} (x - \mu)^2}$	Rms
Kurtosis	$K = \frac{1}{N} \sum_{i=1}^{N} \frac{x_i - \mu^4}{\sigma^4}$	Kurtosis
Skewness	$Sk = \frac{1}{N} \sum_{i=1}^{N} \frac{x_i - \mu^3}{\sigma^3}$	Skewness
Peak value	$x_p = \max_i |x_i|$	Max
Approximate entropy	ApproxEnt $= \O_m - \O_{m+1}$ where, $\O_m = (N - m + 1)^{-1} \sum_{i=1}^{N-m+1} \log(N_i)$	ApproximateEntropy

the approximate entropy and the correlation dimension. We first computed the very basic statistics of signal i.e., mean and standard deviation to check the regularity of signals. Afterwards, in order to get more insight, we extracted impulsive metric i.e. peak value. Impulsive metric helps in analysing the peaks of signal while kurtosis and skewness are higher order statistics which aid in analyzing the behaviour of signals. Finally the non-linear features were calculated in which the approximate entropy checks the amount of unpredictability and the correlation dimension estimates the dimensions of samples. The combination of all theses features helps in finding out the tremor and bradykinesia rhythm. These temporal features were calculated by using equations and Matlab command as illustrated in Table 4.2.

1. **Mean** is the basic statistical parameter for the average value of a signal
2. **Standard deviation** is a value of how far the signal oscillates from the mean. It resembles the average deviation, except the averaging is done with power in place of amplitude.
3. **Root mean square (RMS)** is a measure of the signal's overall energy.
4. **Kurtosis** is a measure of whether the data are heavy-tailed or light-tailed relative to a normal distribution. In short, it estimates relative peakedness of a distribution.
5. **Skewness** demonstrates the symmetry of the probability density function (PDF) of the amplitude of a time series. A time series with an equal number of large and small amplitude values has zero skewness.
6. **Peak value** is the maximum absolute value attained by the signal.
7. **Approximate entropy (ApEn)** measures the unpredictability of fluctuations in time series signals by reconstructing phase space, as presence of repetitive patterns renders in more predictable than a time series in which the patterns are absent.
8. **Correlation dimension** estimates uniformly sampled time domain signal correlation dimension. It is a quantification of dimensionality of space occupied by a set of random points.

Frequency domain features

In frequency domain, first of all, the spectral estimation on time series signals is performed using welch's method by applying hamming window in order to obtain signal spectrum reflecting three dimensional (3D) tremor and bradykinesia movements before extracting spectral domain features. Welch's method is also known as periodogram approach used for estimating power spectra by dividing the time series data into blocks by processing the periodogram in each block. In frequency domain another three features are calculated, which are:

1. **Peak amplitude** of a signal which is the absolute value of its highest intensity, proportional to the energy it sustains.
2. **Peak frequency** quantifies the frequency (period/wavelength) of waves characterized by a peak (maximum energy) in the wave spectrum, sometimes called as the dominant frequency.
3. **Band power** which is seen in the marker function. It counts both power and power spectral density in a specified channel bandwidth.

To extract these features we defined the variable frequency bands with respect to the frequency at which tremor and bradykinesia movements occur.

4.3.3 Classification and Performance

An automated classification system is established to identify tremor and bradykinesia in comparison to age-matched healthy elderly adults. This classification is based on kinematic features and utilizes both unsupervised and supervised machine learning (ML) algorithms. All offline analyses were conducted using MATLAB R2016b (MATLAB, MathWorks, Natick, MA, USA).

Using Unsupervised Method: The Neural Net Clustering Approach

Neural network clustering involves grouping data with shared characteristics into distinct clusters. This technique employs self-organizing maps (SOM). A SOM is constructed using competitive layers that categorize the dataset, organized in the form of feature vectors derived from the collected participant samples. The network undergoes training using the SOM batch algorithm. The map is trained in such a way that each neuron is designated for a specific class. In our case, three classes were classified, for which three neurons were selected, and the performance was assessed using the mean squared error (MSE).

Using Supervised Method: The K-Nearest Neighbors (KNN) Approach

For the automatic evaluation of tremor and bradykinesia in PD patients, we employed the KNN classifier. This non-parametric approach utilizes data to classify new data points based on their proximity and similarity in the feature space.

The main discovery of this research study revolves around identifying the parameters that effectively distinguish instances of tremor and bradykinesia from normal movements. To achieve this, we employed the one-way ANOVA (analysis of variance) test to pinpoint valuable and distinctive features. The outcome of the one-way ANOVA approach is illustrated in Fig. 4.2. Based on the results, features such as approximate entropy, correlation dimension, peak amplitude, and band energies derived from each axis of the accelerometer and the gyroscope demonstrate the highest significance. Consequently, we focused on selecting the features that hold promise in accurately diagnosing tremor and bradykinesia occurrences. These selected features, given their higher rank and importance, serve as strong candidates for training both the NN clustering and KNN models.

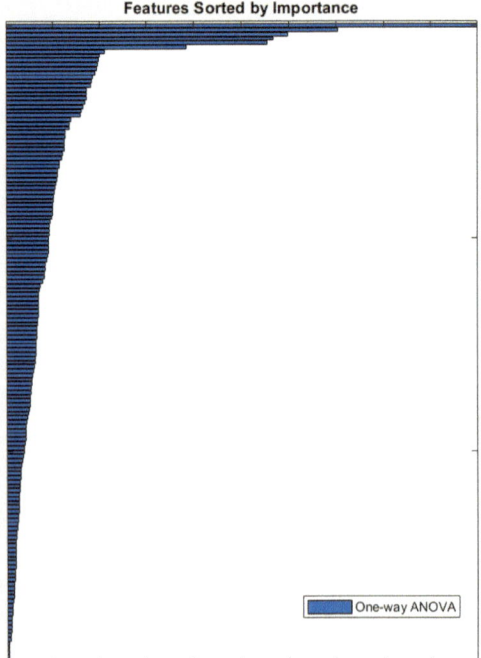

Feature	One-way ANOVA
Sig..._2/ACCZ_ApproxEntropy	254.6353
Sig..._4/GYROY_ApproxEntropy	179.1849
Sig...in/ACCX_ApproxEntropy	152.3177
Sig...in/ACCX_CorrelationDim	144.7471
Sig..._4/GYROY_CorrelationDim	141.1345
Sig...ec/ACCX_BandEnergy	98.2099
Sig...ec/ACCY_PeakAmp8	53.8075
Sig...ec/ACCY_PeakAmp7	51.2424
Sig...ec/ACCX_PeakAmp5	50.6347
Sig...ec/ACCX_PeakAmp6	50.2688
Sig...ec/ACCY_PeakAmp6	49.5595
Sig...ec/ACCX_PeakAmp8	48.7645
Sig..._5/GYROZ_ApproxEntropy	47.5771
Sig...ec/ACCX_PeakAmp7	47.0633
Sig...ec/ACCY_PeakAmp5	46.5709
Sig...ec/ACCZ_BandEnergy	44.2331
Sig...ec/ACCY_PeakAmp4	44.2242
Sig...ec/ACCX_PeakAmp4	43.9375
Sig...ec/ACCX_PeakAmp3	42.9907
Sig...ec/ACCX_PeakAmp2	42.4233
Sig..._5/GYROZ_Kurtosis	41.4022
Sig...ec/ACCY_PeakAmp3	40.8415
Sig...ec/ACCX_PeakAmp1	35.7469
Sig...ec/ACCY_PeakAmp2	34.8464
Sig..._5/GYROZ_CorrelationDim	34.5824
Sig..._5/GYROZ_RMS	32.3681
Sig...ec/ACCY_BandEnergy	32.3057
Sig...ec/ACCX_PeakFreq2	32.2171
Sig...ec/GYROY_BandEnergy	31.8756
Sig..._5/GYROZ_Std	31.7753

Fig. 4.2 Features ranked by significance for the classifiers are presented. On the right side, ANOVA results are shown, while the bars on the left side represent the normalized scores of various features

Table 4.3 Sensitivity and specificity of each class

Class	Sensitivity	Specificity
1 (Healthy)	0.83	1.00
2 (Bradykinesia)	1.00	0.89
3 (Tremor)	1.00	1.00

The KNN trained model yielded results with an accuracy of 91.7%. The choice was made to have 10 neighbors with a hold-out validation of 30%. The sensitivity and specificity of each class are detailed in Table 4.3.

4.4 Deep Learning Based Time-Frequency Features for Parkinson's Severity Assessment

4.4.1 Data Description

The data analyzed in this study is MJFF Levodopa Wearable Sensors Dataset supported by the Michael J. Fox Foundation [5] accessed at www.michaeljfox.org/news/levodopa-response-study. Participants are monitored in-clinic with a sequence of standard activities, as well as at home while carrying out DLAs. The details of patients are given in Table 4.4.

The data collected from the cohort selected for this research study worn Shimmer3 on both upper limbs. However, the data analyzed in this study come from the most affected upper limb of the patients. These wearables were worn by subjects for a duration of 4 days.

- On Day 1 of data collection, subjects were present in laboratory in ON state (after taking medication(s)), answered demographic as well as medical history questions, completed sections I, II, and IV of MDS-UPDRS and donned the wearable devices. Then, they carry out section III of the MDS-UPDRS and ADL. The list of activities performed includes standing, walking in straight line for 30 s with and without backward counting, walking upstairs, walking downstairs, walking through narrow corridor, finger to nose for 15 s, alternating hand movements for 15 s, drawing, typing on each keyboard for 30 s, opening a bottle and pouring water (3 times), arranging sheets of paper in a folder, assembling nuts and bolts for 30 s, folding a towel three times and sitting. For each instance of each performed task, clinical labels of symptom severity or presence were provided by the observer. The labeled symptoms were tremor, bradykinesia and dyskinesia (rates 0–4).
- During Days 2 and 3, the participants performed their usual free body activities wearing all the sensors. Shimmer subjects were also asked to perform a sequence of standard tasks corresponding to specific items of section III of MDS-UPDRS such as alternating hand movements for 30 s (once for each arm), finger to nose

Table 4.4 Demographic details of PD patients

Patient	Gender	Age	Dominant hand	Most effected side
3BOS	Female	86	Right	Right
4BOS	Female	52	Right	Right
5BOS	Male	74	Right	Right
6BOS	Male	62	Right	Left
7BOS	Male	74	Right	Right
8BOS	Male	64	Right	Right
9BOS	Female	69	Right	Left
10BOS	Male	83	Right	Right
11BOS	Male	61	Right	Right
12BOS	Female	82	Right	Right
13BOS	Male	68	Right	Right
14BOS	Male	65	Right	Right
15BOS	Female	70	Right	Right
16BOS	Male	70	Right	Bilateral
17BOS	Female	60	Left	Bilateral
18BOS	Male	65	Right	Right
19BOS	Male	77	Right	Right

for 30 s and sitting quietly for 30 s every 30 min, for total of 7 times on each of the two days at home.

- On Day 4, the participants came to laboratory in OFF state and withheld for around 12 h. The same procedure of Day 1 has been followed once again on Day 4. Initially, the motor tasks were performed in OFF state. Following that, the subjects took their regularly scheduled morning medication dose, and performed 5–7 repetitions of the motor tasks with the same timeline of Day 1 (every 30 min). Severity scores and symptom presence/ absence were assessed again. Finally, the subjects doffed the sensors.

For each instance of each task performed, clinical labels of symptom severity and/or symptom presence were provided by a clinician. The severity scores of tremor (0–4) and bradykinesia (0–4) along with symptoms presence or absence are provided for Day 1 and Day 4. In order to estimate severity of tremor and bradykinesia we analyzed the data of patients from Day 1 and Day 4 only.

Comparison of Data Collected From A-WEAR Bracelet and From Shimmer Device

Due to the heightened vulnerability of older individuals, particularly those with underlying medical conditions, to contracting severe illnesses amid the COVID-19 pandemic, our study was precluded from creating a dataset sourced directly from Parkinson's disease (PD) patients. Consequently, we opted to juxtapose data originating from the Shimmer unit with data derived from the proposed bracelet. The accelerometer embedded in the Shimmer device captures data akin to our dataset. To validate our approach, we obtained parallel data from a single patient using both the Shimmer device and our bracelet while adhering to COVID-19 safety protocols.

The two recordings exhibit an almost identical resemblance in terms of 6-digit numeric values and sample rates. In the Shimmer device scenario, the sampling frequency was set at 100 Hz, a rate that can also be configured for the A-WEAR bracelet. Notably, the accelerometers' noise in both cases—both the Shimmer device and the A-WEAR bracelet—was extremely minimal and exerted no discernible impact on the datasets. This underscores the remarkable compatibility of the dataset collected by the Michael J. Fox Foundation, utilizing wearable sensors [5], with the proposed computational technique's validation process.

As in Table 4.5 we know their is a subject of imbalanced distribution of data or the lack of class density in data. Therefore, in this section we proposed a strategy to classify imbalanced RT severity dataset by adapting resampling techniques. The findings of our previous work [6] shows oversampling techniques work better than undersampling and hybrid sampling technique. Based on the extensive literature review, our research work adopted a feature extraction method over raw data for Parkinson's disease (PD) assessment. The findings from the literature review indicate a prevalent preference among researchers for the feature extraction approach over scalograms. This preference can be attributed to several reasons. Firstly, scalograms, as representations of signals in the time-frequency domain, may introduce a certain degree of information loss during the transformation process. In contrast, extracting features directly from raw signals enables the preservation of the complete information contained within the original data. Secondly, feature extraction from raw signals provides greater flexibility in selecting and designing specific features tailored to the

Table 4.5 Imbalanced data distribution

Class (Tremor severity)	Instances	After oversampling
0	2479	2479
1	1504	2479
2	464	2479
3	172	2479
4	90	2479
Total	4709	12395

unique characteristics of the data and the requirements of the classification task. This adaptability allows researchers to capture relevant patterns and dynamics specific to Parkinson's disease more effectively. Additionally, while scalograms often generate high-dimensional feature representations that can be computationally expensive and require further dimensionality reduction techniques, feature extraction from raw signals can potentially yield lower-dimensional feature representations. This not only improves the efficiency of the subsequent classification task but also enhances its interpretability. Features extracted directly from raw signals are more readily interpretable, as they correspond to specific physiological or biomechanical aspects of PD. This interpretability plays a crucial role in deepening our understanding of the underlying mechanisms and contributing valuable insights to the clinical domain.

While scalograms or time-frequency mapping can provide valuable insights into the time-frequency characteristics of Parkinson's disease signals, DL approaches offer a more comprehensive and automated solution by extracting high-level features directly from the raw data, leading to improved classification performance and robustness.

4.4.2 Cloud Service: Data Processing and Decision Making

Figure 4.3 explains the pipeline of data processing inside the cloud. First, the accelerometer data from wearable device uploaded to the cloud in form of CSV file. The recorded signals are labelled and filtered out after that using band pass filter. In the second step, the set of tremor severity features in time and frequency domain are extracted from the preprocessed samples. In the third step, data is segregated into training and test subsets. Additionally, to avoid classifier bias training, the data is resampled. The data distribution is based on 10-fold cross validation. Finally, tremor severity levels (0–4) are estimated by passing training and test data into CatBoost classifier. After training and testing the results are updated on web and mobile app. The registered doctor can then recommend the treatment and advice on cloud platform. The report and results can also be accessed by patients. Each step is described in details in the subsequent sections.

Signal Processing

The experimental protocol involved two visits to the study site, as previously detailed in Sect. 4.4.1. During each visit (both in ON and OFF states), subjects were assigned a set of tasks to complete. These tasks, sourced from the motor assessment component of the MDS-UPDRS Part III and encompassing Activities of Daily Living (ADLs), were chosen to enable the classification of these tasks. ADLs were selected due to their demand for both overall mobility (such as carrying a book) and fine motor skills (like writing a sentence), which mirror real-world scenarios. The assessment

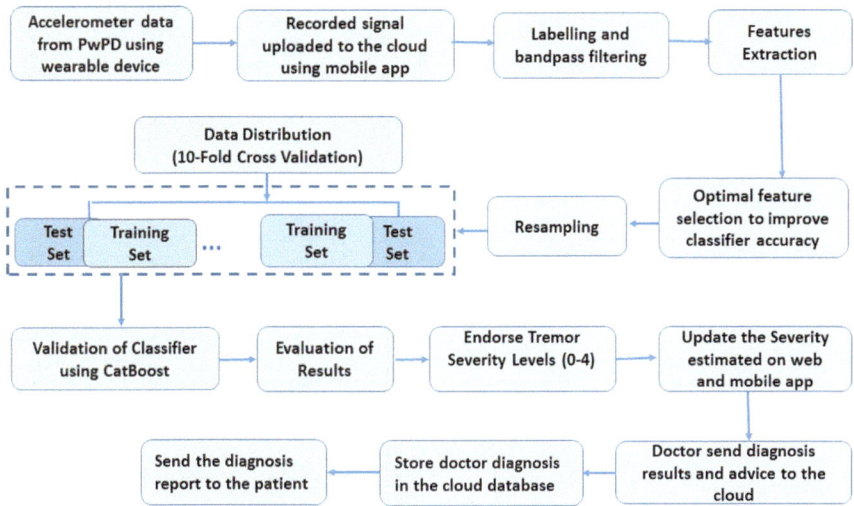

Fig. 4.3 Pipeline of data processing inside cloud

was overseen by a neurosurgeon who assigned grades ranging from 0 to 4 to the items.

The data encompassed five primary levels of severity, offering comprehensive coverage. Initial data processing involved segmenting the raw signal into individual motion events using a JAVA script, with a 3 s temporal window preceding motion onset. The choice of a 3 s window for the tremor classifier was grounded in prior research within the domains of PD symptom monitoring and human activity recognition. This window duration has proven to provide adequate resolution for extracting relevant time and frequency domain features [7, 8]. The 3 s length is apt for capturing signal attributes associated with high-frequency movements, given that tremors usually exhibit fundamental frequencies between 3 and 12 Hz. However, a window length of at least 1–2 s is essential to strike a balance between classification accuracy and inference speed [8].

Subsequently, the raw sensor data undergoes band-pass filtering using a second-order Butterworth IIR filter, employing cutoff frequencies of 3–12 Hz. This step attenuates all frequency components outside the tremor range. Figure 4.4 depicts the analysis of filtered data across various severity scores. The coefficient of variation of the filtered signal is then subjected to an empirically developed threshold to detect hand movement. This procedure is reiterated for accurate identification of hand movement.

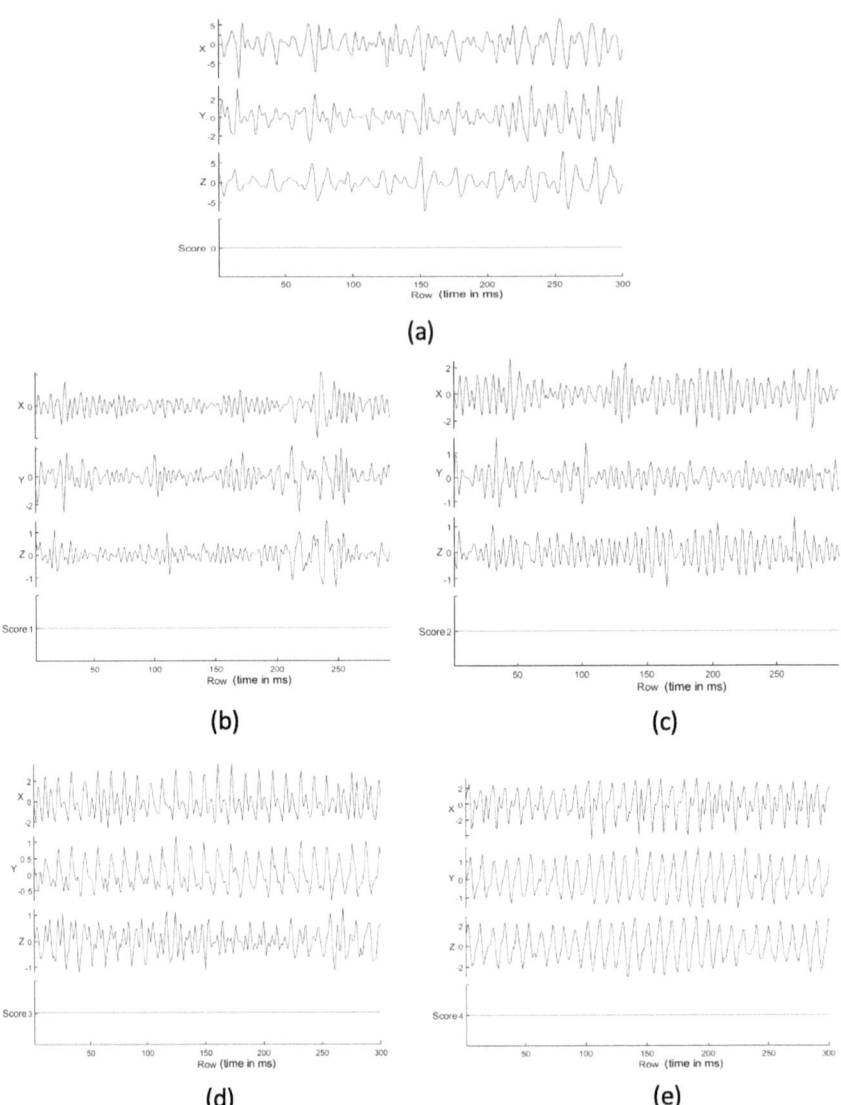

Fig. 4.4 Analysis of Accelerometer signals for each severity level

4.4.3   Features Extraction and Selection

Consistency and amplitude are the two metrics used to evaluate resting tremor. While amplitude gauges the speed and size of tremor-related movements, consistency assesses the proportion of time that tremor is present. Using prior research as a guide, a set of features crucial for analyzing of tremors were retrieved from the filtered signals. Firstly, we divide the signal into 3 s windows and extract the respective features for each window. However, the frequency domain features are extracted after converting the raw signal from the time domain to the frequency domain using the Fast Fourier Transform (FFT), according to Expression (4.1) below, Table 4.6 presents a list of the extracted features along with a description of each.

$$F(y) = \sum_{t=0}^{W_l - 1} x_t e^{\frac{-j2\lambda yt}{W_l}} \tag{4.1}$$

for $y = 0, \ldots, W_l - 1$. $F(y)$ is a complex series is a complex series which has the identical dimensions as the input sequence $(x_t)_{t=0}^{W_l}$ and $e^{\frac{-j2\lambda yt}{W_l}}$ is a primitive Nth root of unity. The extracted features were acquired by processing the acceleration values of X-, Y-, and Z-axis. The features extracted from motion signals that differentiates tremor and its severity levels are: mean, maximum, minimum, variance, root mean square (RMS) kurtosis, skewness, power, covariance, standard deviation etc. in time and frequency domains. Similar to this, a prior study revealed that frequency sub-bands and tremor severity are strongly connected [9], since each tremor severity or score only occurs within a certain frequency range and therefore the sum of total band power, relative spectral peak per band and so on are extracted.

After features extraction, we performed feature selection which is very important for model building. Feature selection is performed using **FeatureWiz** python library. Using featurewiz library, the best features in the dataset of any size can be easily found, [10]. It utilizes two distinct methodologies that together aid in identifying the best features. These techniques are:

- SULOV: SULOV is an acronym for Searching for Uncorrelated List of Variables. This method is utilized to pinpoint pairs of variables that surpass a pre defined correlation threshold, signifying a robust association between them. Once these variable pairings are determined, the Mutual Information Score (MIS) is employed to quantify the extent of information that can be gleaned from one random variable when another is known. This calculation is conducted subsequent to the identification of these variable pairs.

  Following this, the approach takes into account the pair of variables exhibiting the lowest correlation and the highest MIS scores, which are subsequently subjected to further processing.
- Recursive XGBoost: The variables selected through the SULOV technique undergo a recursive XGBoost procedure. This entails utilizing XGBoost to iteratively process these variables, creating smaller datasets derived from the original dataset. This iterative process aids in pinpointing the most suitable features for the target variable.

  In this process, the algorithm identifies the top feature variables within the dataset. Consequently, Featurewiz effectively establishes associations between various variables by considering their MIS scores and correlations with distinct feature variables.

Table 4.6 Features extracted from accelerometer data

Features and Abbreviations	Domain	Formula
Mean ($\bar{X}$)	T	$\bar{X} = \frac{1}{N} \sum_{i=1}^{N} x_i$
Maximum (MAX)	T	$MAX = \max(x_i)$
Peak (P_m)	T	$P_m = \max(|x_i|)$
Root Mean Square (RMS)	T and F	$RMS = \sqrt{\frac{1}{N} \sum_{i=1}^{N} x_i^2}$
Variance (VAR)	T	$VAR = \frac{\sum_{i=1}^{N} (x_i - \bar{x})^2}{N-1}$
kurtosis (KURT)	T	$KURT = \frac{1}{N} \sum^{N} (\frac{x_i - \bar{x}}{\sigma})^4$
Skewness (SKEW)	T	$SKEW = \frac{N}{(N-1)(N-2)} \sum (\frac{x_i - \bar{x}}{\sigma})^3$
Power (POW)	T and F	$POW = \frac{1}{N} \sum_{i=1}^{N} x_i^2$
Standard deviation (σ)	T and F	$\sigma = \sqrt{\frac{\sum_{i=1}^{n} (x_i - \varphi)^2}{n-1}}$
Minimum (MIN)	T and F	$MIN = \min(x_i)$
Covariance (Cov)	T and F	$Cov_{(x,y)} = S_{xy} = \frac{\sum_{i=1}^{n} (x_i - \bar{x})(y_i - \bar{y})}{n-1}$
Mean of band power spectrum (S_μ)	F	$S_\mu = \frac{1}{n} \sum_{i=1}^{n} S(f)_i$
Max of band power spectrum (S_{MAX})	F	$S_{MAX} = \max S(f)_i$
Sum of total band power (S_{SBP})	F	$S_{SBP} = \sum_{i=1}^{n} S(f)_i$
Variance of band power (S_v)	F	$S_v = \frac{\sum_{i=1}^{n} (S(f)_i - S_\mu)^2}{n-1}$
Skewness of band power (S_s)	F	$S_s = \frac{\frac{1}{n} \sum_{i=1}^{n} (S(f)_i - S_\mu)^3}{S_v^{\frac{3}{2}}}$
Kurtosis of band power (S_k)	F	$S_k = \frac{\frac{1}{n} \sum_{i=1}^{n} (S(f)_i - S_\mu)^4}{S_v^{\frac{4}{2}}}$
Relative spectral peak per band (S_{RSPPB})	F	$S_{RSPPB} = \frac{\max(S(f)_i)}{\frac{1}{n} \sum_{i=1}^{n} S(f)_i}$

Resampling method

The dataset which we analyzed in this research is imbalance. Imbalanced data is one when there is an uneven distribution of samples across class labels. Since all classes are equally important in classification problem. The details of sample distribution in each class is mentioned in Table 4.7. According to the results we achieved in our previous research study [11], oversampling methods gave better results in terms of accuracy and IBA_α than undersampling and hybrid sampling. Because of this, we adopted oversampling techniques in this study.

In order to make the number of instances in the minority class more closely resemble or match the number of examples in the majority classes, oversampling is the process of replicating or synthesizing additional examples of the minority classes. Oversampling techniques are frequently used by researchers because they

Table 4.7 Imbalanced data distribution

Class (Tremor severity)	Instances	After oversampling
0	2479	2479
1	1504	2479
2	464	2479
3	172	2479
4	90	2479
Total	4709	12395

can balance class distributions without excluding potentially important majority cases [12]. The dataset is initially partitioned into k stratified divisions, and within the cross-validation process, oversampling is exclusively applied to the training set, which corresponds to $k - 1$ partitions. This approach ensures that oversampling does not affect the model or introduce exposure to test set patterns during training. As a result, an unbiased estimation of the model's generalization capability from the training data can be achieved.

The intention behind this condition is to prevent overoptimism, a phenomenon that arises when identical or highly similar patterns exist in both the training and test sets [13]. In such cases (referred to as "CV after Oversampling"), the model's performance in the test sets becomes indistinguishable from its performance in the training sets. The presence of comparable patterns in both partitions obstructs the model's ability to effectively generalize to new, unseen data. Overoptimism is particularly associated with flawed implementations of the cross-validation technique when oversampling is applied.

1. SMOTE: The Synthetic Minority Oversampling TEchnique, known as SMOTE, is a widely utilized approach for generating new samples, as introduced by Chawla et al. in their work [14]. SMOTE employs a k-nearest neighbor approach to create synthetic data. The process commences by randomly selecting data points from the minority class, followed by identifying their k-nearest neighbors. The synthetic data is then formed by combining these k-nearest neighbor data points with randomly selected data points. This technique is particularly beneficial for generating synthetic data when dealing with continuous features and classification problems.

2. Borderline SMOTE: Borderline-SMOTE is a modified version of the SMOTE technique. Unlike SMOTE, which introduces synthetic data randomly between the two classes, Borderline-SMOTE specifically generates synthetic data along the decision boundary separating the two classes. This targeted approach aims to enhance the minority class representation by focusing on the borderline instances. Figure 4.5 shows the difference between without oversampling data with over-resampling techniques i.e. SMOTE Borderline.

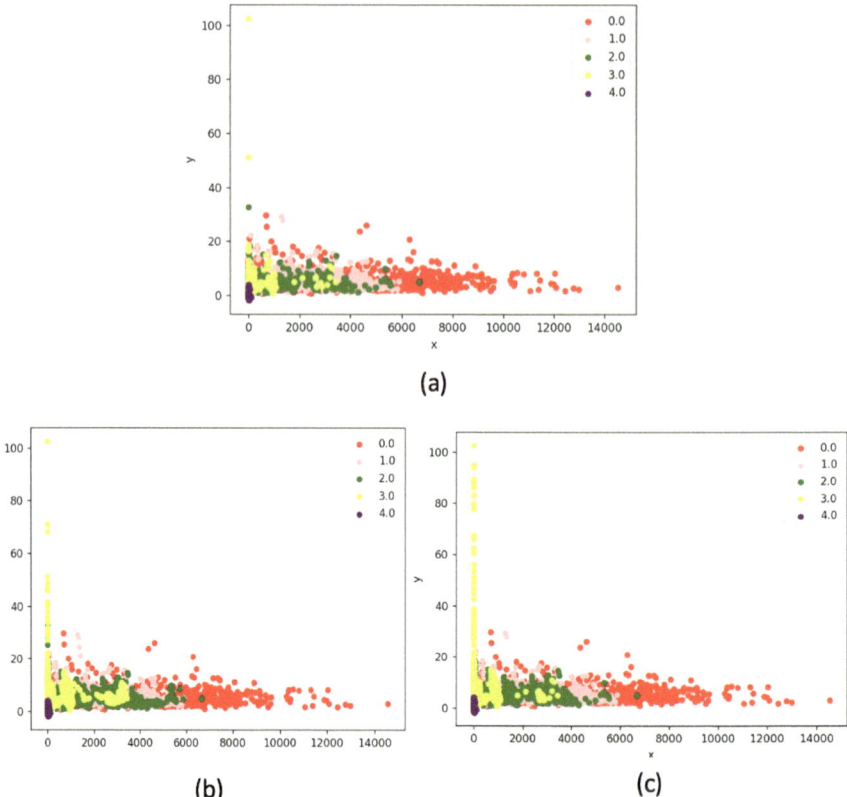

Fig. 4.5 This figure illustrates the difference of before and after over-resampling, **a** is data without resampling, **b** is data after applying Smote overresampling method, **c** is data after applying Borderline Smote overresampling method

Classifier

The term 'CatBoost' is a combination of the phrases 'Category' and 'Boosting'. It is an open-source machine learning (gradient boosting) method [15]. It was created in 2017 by Yandex. The key feature is that it generates balanced (symmetric) trees, in contrast to XGBoost and LightGBM. The same condition is used to divide the leaves from the preceding tree at each stage. For each of the level's nodes, the feature-split pair that accounts the least loss is chosen. This balanced tree architecture helps with effective CPU implementation, cuts down on prediction time, creates quick model implementers, and reduces overfitting because the structure acts as regularization. Unlike other classic boosting algorithms, CatBoost employs the idea of ordered boosting, a permutation-driven method, to train the model on a portion of data while computing residuals on a different subset, preventing target leakage and overfitting.

Meanwhile, the prediction time of CatBoost came out to be faster than XGBoost and LightGBM; which is extremely important for low latency environments.

Considering these factors of CatBoost and other intelligent techniques for finding the best features in a given model, we adopted CatBoost classifier to estimate severity level of tremors in PwPD based on the data collected from wearable device. The important parameters that we set for our model are: $iterations = 1000$, $loss_function = $ 'MultiClass', $bootstrap_type = $ 'Bayesian', $eval_metric = $ 'MultiClass', $leaf\_estimation\_iterations = 100$, $random\_strength = 0.5$, depth $= 7$, $learning\_rate = 0.1$, $bagging\_temperature = 0.5$, $task_type = $ 'GPU'.

Instead of using a straightforward train/test split, cross-validation is a common technique to improve a model's accuracy. The cross-validation process involves randomly rearranging the data set, dividing it into k groups, using a subset of the data as a test set while using the remaining data to build a model and determine its accuracy, and then calculating and reporting the mean of all k obtained accuracy. If the value for k is assigned to be the number of observations, then it is called leave-one-out cross-validation. It turns out that CatBoost with $k = 10$ folds gives the best accuracy, approximately 96%. Figure 4.6 displays the accuracy scores of CatBoost with $K - fold$ validation using ROC curve and Confusion matrix.

4.5 Results and Discussions

Tables 4.8 and 4.9 show the best results obtained from the CatBoost classifer in combination with SMOTE and Borderline SMOTE resampling techniques. Among these results, the best performance obtained with SMOTE achieved 96% overall accuracy. Accuracy, precision, sensitivity (True Positive Rate), and specificity (True Negative Rate) are the commonly employed metrics for assessing the classification algorithms' performance. Nonetheless, when dealing with imbalanced classification problems, relying solely on these metrics can be misleading and inadequate as they can be impacted by the distribution of data. As a result, this study incorporates advanced metrics beyond the conventional ones, such as precision, F1- score, sensitivity, specificity, G-mean and the index of balanced accuracy (IBA). The following metrics are calculated using the following formulas:

$$Accuracy = \frac{TP + TN}{TP + TN + FP + FN} \tag{4.2}$$

$$Precision = \frac{TP}{TP + FP} \tag{4.3}$$

$$Sensitivity = TPR = \frac{TP}{TP + FN} \tag{4.4}$$

Table 4.8 Performance metrics of CatBoost classifier with SMOTE technique

SMOTE	Score 0	Score 1	Score 2	Score 3	Score 4	Overall
Accuracy	0.96	0.98	0.98	0.99	1	0.96
Precision	0.99	0.96	0.95	0.92	1.00	0.96
F1-score	0.97	0.97	0.92	0.96	1.00	0.96
Sensitivity	0.94	0.97	0.98	1	1	0.97
Specificity	0.98	0.98	0.98	0.99	1	0.98
IBA_α	1.0	0.99	1.0	1.0	1.0	0.99
Gmean	0.95	0.97	0.98	0.99	1.0	0.97

Table 4.9 Performance metrics of CatBoost classifier with Borderline SMOTE

Borderline-SMOTE	Score 0	Score 1	Score 2	Score 3	Score 4	Overall
Accuracy	0.97	0.92	0.96	0.97	0.97	0.95
Precision	0.99	0.97	0.88	0.96	1.0	0.96
F1-score	0.97	0.98	0.92	0.96	1.0	0.96
Sensitivity	0.95	0.98	0.97	0.96	1	0.97
Specificity	0.98	0.98	0.98	0.99	1	0.98
IBA_α	0.99	0.96	0.97	1	1	0.98
Gmean	0.96	0.98	0.97	0.97	1	0.97

$$Specificity = TNR = \frac{TN}{TN + FP} \tag{4.5}$$

$$F1 = \frac{2 \times Precision \times Sensitivity}{Precision + Sensitivity} \tag{4.6}$$

$$Gmean = \sqrt{Sensitivity \times Specificity} \tag{4.7}$$

$$IBA_\alpha = 1 + \alpha \times (TPR - TNR) \times GMean^2, \text{ where } 0 \leq \alpha \leq 1 \tag{4.8}$$

where TP, FP, TN, FN, TPR, TNR, and α, refer respectively to, true positive, false positive, true negative, false negative, true positive rate, true negative rate, and weighting factor. Comparing the results of both resampling techniques it is evident both oversampling methods give good results but SMOTE technique gave better results not just with accuracy but in terms of overall IBA and accuracy.

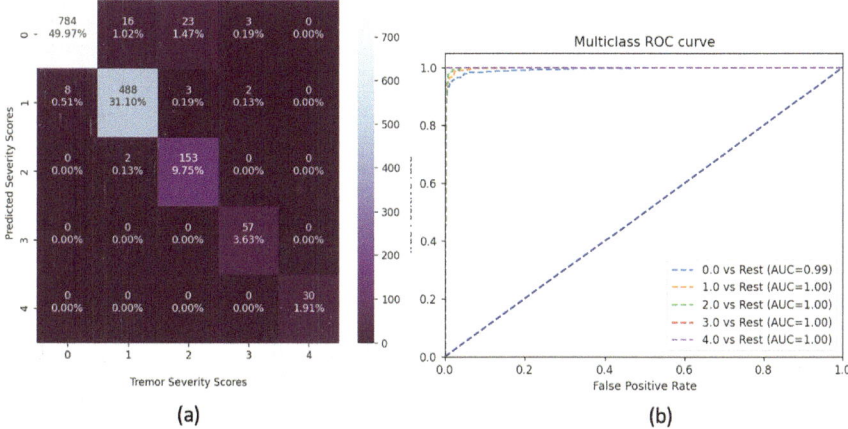

Fig. 4.6 Confusion matrix and ROC curve using CATBoost classifier in combination with SMOTE oversampling method

Figure 4.6 shows the performance of CatBoost classifer, on PD tremor severity dataset resampled using over-sampling technique. Figure 4.6a shows the confusion matrix of CatBoost classifer using SMOTE over-resampling technoique.

We calculated Receiver Operating Characteristic (ROC) metric to evaluate the classifier output quality. The effectiveness of the model may be estimated using the ROC area under curve (AUC) metric. Although, this metric accurately depicts relative changes in model performance, it might be too optimistic for datasets with extreme imbalance. Two axes are typically included on ROC curves: an X axis for false positive rate and a Y axis for true positive rate. Therefore, the 'optimal' placement is in the upper left corner of the plot, which has a false positive rate of 0 and a true positive rate of 1. Although, this is not very practical, it does suggest that a larger region beneath the curve (AUC) is often desirable. ROC curves are frequently used in binary classification to examine a classifier's performance. It is important to binarize the data in order to expand the ROC curve and ROC area to multi-label classification. It is possible to create one ROC curve per label, but it is also possible to construct ROC curves by treating each member of the label indicator matrix as a binary prediction (micro-averaging).

Macro-averaging, which equally weighs the categorization of each label, is another assessment metric for multi-label classification. Since CatBoost classifier in a combination of SMOTE resampling technique gives better results i.e. 96% accuracy. The ROC curve of this multiclass problem is shown in Fig. 4.6. However, the extended metrics one-vs-one ROC AUC scores are 0.99 (macro) and 0.98 (weighted by prevalence). While, one-vs-rest ROC AUC scores are 0.998 (macro) and 0.996 (weighted by prevalence).

The proposed closed-based system is the answer for PD patient's continuous home monitoring and evaluation with a correct diagnosis and severity estimation. To prove the correct marking and the levodopa dosage, we used the accelerometer

Table 4.10 Comparison with the state-of-the-art

Refs.	Measured symptoms	Sensor	Approach	Results	Severity score (s)
Rigas et al. [16]	Tremor	Accelerometer	Time and frequency domain features classified with HMM	Accuracy = 87%, specificity = 85%, sensitivity = 0.85, precision = 0.66	0, 1, 2, 3
Sigcha et al. [17]	Tremor	Accelerometer	290 features extracted and classified using AdaBoost	Specificity = 86%, Sensitivity = 86%, AUC=93%	0, 1, 2
Dai et al. [18]	Tremor	Gyroscope, Magnetometer, Accelerometer	Features extracted and classified with an SVM model	Accuracy = 96%, Specificity = 100%, Sensitivity =97%	–
Kim et al. [19]	Tremor	Gyroscope, Accelerometer	2D image representation for CNN model using sensor signals	Accuracy = 85%, Sensitivity = 79%, Precision = 81%, Kappa coefficient = 85%, Correlation coefficient = 93%	0, 1, 2, (3, 4)
This work	Tremor and Bradykinesia	Accelerometer	Raw data transformed and classified with AlexNet	Tremor: Accuracy = 9 0.9%, Gmean = 0.94, IBA_α = 0.93 Bradykinesia: Accuracy = 86.4%, Gmean = 0.916, IBA_α = 0.91	Severities 0, 1, 2, 3, 4

data from PwPD using Shimmer device, the data being collected by Michael J.Fox foundation. The data is labeled into two phases i.e., when the patients took their medicine on time (ON state) and when patients missed their medicine (OFF state) and performed activities. Compared to the previous research studies and systems, in this proposed model we adopted the part of hand-crafted feature extraction and feature selection method and performed resampling over the data. For severity estimation, we employed deep learning (DL) based model which is CatBoost classifier.

The model is trained for tremor severity score analysis. CatBoost model shows very promising results by giving 96% accuracy for tremor with good performance in terms of sensitivity and specificity in each scoring class. Table 4.10 shows the summary results and comparison with the state-of-the-art. The measured cardinal motor symptoms, the sensors attached, ML or DL approach for analysis, the evaluation metrics and measured severities are explained in the table. High classification performance was obtained in [18] but this study did not work on all levels of severity. Similarly the studies [16–18] extracted number of features and performed feature selection step in which there is risk of missing important features. Only the study [19] employed 2D image representation of inertial data and implemented CNN classification model but the accuracy is 85% which is less. So, most of the studies did not take into consideration to measure tremor along all levels or types of severities.

References

1. *Parkinson's Disease Exam*, Stanford Medicine 25, https://stanfordmedicine25.stanford.edu/the25/parkinsondisease.html [Accessed 2023/09/25 17:25:31].
2. *Neurological tremor: sensors, signal processing and emerging applications*, Giuliana Grimaldi and Mario Manto, *Sensors*, vol. 10, no. 2, pp. 1399–1422, 2010, Molecular Diversity Preservation International.
3. *Handbook of tremor disorders*, Leslie J Findley and William C Koller, vol. 30, 1994, Informa Health Care.
4. D. Pan, R. Dhall, A. Lieberman, and D. B. Petitti, "A mobile cloud-based Parkinson's disease assessment system for home-based monitoring," *JMIR mHealth and uHealth*, vol. 3, no. 1, pp. e3956, 2015.
5. Sage Bionetworks MJFF Levodopa Wearable Sensors Dataset. (https://www.synapse.org/#!Synapse:syn20681023/wiki/594678 [Accessed September 4, 2023],2019)
6. Channa, A., Cramariuc, O., Memon, M., Popescu, N., Mammone, N. & Ruggeri, G. Parkinson's disease resting tremor severity classification using machine learning with resampling techniques. *Frontiers In Neuroscience*. **16** pp. 955464–955464 (2022)
7. Patel, S., Lorincz, K., Hughes, R., Huggins, N., Growdon, J., Standaert, D., Akay, M., Dy, J., Welsh, M. & Bonato, P. Monitoring motor fluctuations in patients with Parkinson's disease using wearable sensors. *IEEE Transactions On Information Technology In Biomedicine*. **13**, 864–873 (2009)
8. Banos, O., Galvez, J., Damas, M., Pomares, H. & Rojas, I. Window size impact in human activity recognition. *Sensors*. **14**, 6474–6499 (2014)
9. Niazmand, K., Tonn, K., Kalaras, A., Kammermeier, S., Boetzel, K., Mehrkens, J. & Lueth, T. A measurement device for motion analysis of patients with parkinson's disease using sensor based smart clothes. *2011 5th International Conference On Pervasive Computing Technologies For Healthcare (PervasiveHealth) And Workshops*. pp. 9–16 (2011)

10. AutoViML AutoViML/featurewiz: Use Advanced Feature Engineering Strategies and select best features from your data set with a single line of code.. *GitHub*. (2020)
11. Channa, A., Memon, M., Cramariuc, O., Popescu, N., Mammone, N. & Ruggeri, G. Parkinson's Disease Resting Tremor Severity Classification using Machine Learning with Resampling Techniques. *Frontiers In Neuroscience*. pp. 1664
12. Haixiang, G., Yijing, L., Shang, J., Mingyun, G., Yuanyue, H. & Bing, G. Learning from class-imbalanced data: Review of methods and applications. *Expert Systems With Applications*. **73** pp. 220–239 (2017)
13. Santos, M., Soares, J., Abreu, P., Araujo, H. & Santos, J. Cross-validation for imbalanced datasets: avoiding overoptimistic and overfitting approaches [research frontier]. *Ieee ComputatioNal INtelligeNCe MagaziNe*.
14. Chawla, N., Bowyer, K., Hall, L. & Kegelmeyer, W. SMOTE: synthetic minority over-sampling technique. *Journal Of Artificial Intelligence Research*. **16** pp. 321–357 (2002)
15. Dorogush, A., Ershov, V. & Gulin, A. CatBoost: gradient boosting with categorical features support. ArXiv Preprint ArXiv:1810.11363. (2018)
16. G. Rigas, A. Tzallas, M. G. Tsipouras, P. Bougia, E. E. Tripoliti, D. Baga, D. I. Fotiadis, S. G. Tsouli, and S. Konitsiotis, "Assessment of tremor activity in the Parkinson's disease using a set of wearable sensors," *IEEE Transactions on Information Technology in Biomedicine*, vol. 16, no. 3, pp. 478–487, 2012.
17. L. Sigcha, I. Pavón, N. Costa, S. Costa, M. Gago, P. Arezes, J. M. López, and G. De Arcas, "Automatic resting tremor assessment in Parkinson's disease using smartwatches and multitask convolutional neural networks," *Sensors*, vol. 21, no. 1, pp. 291, 2021.
18. H. Dai, G. Cai, Z. Lin, Z. Wang, and Q. Ye, "Validation of inertial sensing-based wearable device for tremor and bradykinesia quantification," *IEEE Journal of Biomedical and Health Informatics*, vol. 25, no. 4, pp. 997–1005, 2020.
19. H. B. Kim, W. W. Lee, A. Kim, H. J. Lee, H. Y. Park, H. S. Jeon, S. K. Kim, B. Jeon, and K. S. Park, "Wrist sensor-based tremor severity quantification in Parkinson's disease using convolutional neural network," *Computers in biology and medicine*, vol. 95, pp. 140–146, 2018.

Chapter 5
Transforming Parkinson's Disease Care: Cloud Service Empowered by ServiceNow Technology

Abstract This chapter introduces a cloud-based service leveraging ServiceNow technology for the management and analysis of accelerometer data collected via a specially designed bracelet worn by PD patients. The chapter delineates the seamless flow of data from the bracelet to a mobile app and then to the ServiceNow platform, where it is securely stored and processed. It elaborates on the integration of a DL module within the ServiceNow platform, enabling continuous data processing and result updates. These updated results are made accessible through both a web application and a mobile app, ensuring convenience and accessibility for patients, healthcare professionals, and the broader PD community. The cloud-based nature of the service guarantees scalability, security, and effortless updates. Overall, this chapter serves as a testament to the successful implementation of a cloud service employing ServiceNow technology to benefit PD patients.

5.1 Cloud Service

5.1.1 The ServiceNow Platform

It's important to note that ServiceNow is primarily known as an IT Service Management (ITSM) platform, and while it offers customization and integration capabilities, DL and complex data processing are not its primary focus. You may need to leverage external libraries, frameworks, or cloud services for the deep learning aspects while utilizing ServiceNow for its workflow automation, data storage, and user interface capabilities.

ServiceNow is a platform-as-a-service provider, offering technical management support, such as IT service management, to the IT operations of large corporations, including help desk functionality. Even though its main purpose is to satisfy the IT workflows of business companies, it offers (i) a top infrastructure for cloud applications with out-of-the-box infrastructure for fast databases, (ii) the possibility to develop JavaScript applications on top of it with easy support for adding REST API methods for third party tools (or in our case the bracelet), (iii) it also allows other kind of application like Java, PowerShell, etc. to run on a local machine and fetch

© The Author(s), under exclusive license to Springer Nature Switzerland AG 2024   51
A. Channa and N. Popescu, *Deep Learning in Smart eHealth Systems*,
SpringerBriefs in Computer Science, https://doi.org/10.1007/978-3-031-45003-7_5

the results to the cloud and (iv) offers free instances for developers that want to experiment with the platform. To use ServiceNow for building a web application that integrates wearable device data, stores it, processes it using DL algorithms, and produces results, one can follow these general steps:

- Data collection from wearable devices: Connect the wearable devices to ServiceNow using appropriate protocols and APIs. This can involve using technologies like Bluetooth, Wi-Fi, or specialized APIs provided by the wearable device manufacturer. Retrieve the data from the devices and send it to ServiceNow for further processing.
- Data storage in ServiceNow: ServiceNow provides a robust database and storage capabilities. Create a data model in ServiceNow to define the structure and attributes of the wearable device data. Use ServiceNow's tables and fields to store the incoming data in a structured manner. This ensures that the data is securely stored and easily accessible for processing.
- Deep learning algorithm integration: Develop or import your deep learning algorithm for processing the wearable device data. You can use popular deep learning frameworks like TensorFlow or PyTorch. Integrate the algorithm into your web application within the ServiceNow platform. This can involve developing custom scripts or using ServiceNow integration capabilities to connect with the algorithm.
- Data processing with deep learning: Use the stored wearable device data from ServiceNow as input for your deep learning algorithm. Process the data using the algorithm to generate the desired results. This can include classification, prediction, anomaly detection, or any other task that your deep learning model is designed to perform.
- Result storage and visualization: Store the results generated by the deep learning algorithm back in ServiceNow. Define appropriate fields or tables in ServiceNow to capture and store the output. Additionally, create visualization components within your web application using ServiceNow's UI capabilities to present the results to users in a meaningful way.
- Continuous data processing: Set up processes or workflows within ServiceNow to handle the continuous flow of wearable device data. This can involve automating data ingestion, processing, and result generation on a regular basis or in real-time. Implement scheduling or event-based triggers to ensure timely processing of new data as it arrives.
- Security and access control: As wearable device data may contain sensitive information, implement security measures within ServiceNow to protect the data. Define access controls, encryption, and other security protocols to ensure that only authorized individuals can access and process the data.

Given these inherent benefits, it's evident that this platform could serve as an intermediary or bridge connecting the bracelet and the DL computational method. Leveraging ServiceNow, we can establish a POST method atop the platform or utilize the readily available built-in options to transmit the collected data to a designated database table. This setup enables a script to retrieve the data through a GET method and subsequently input them into the DL algorithm.

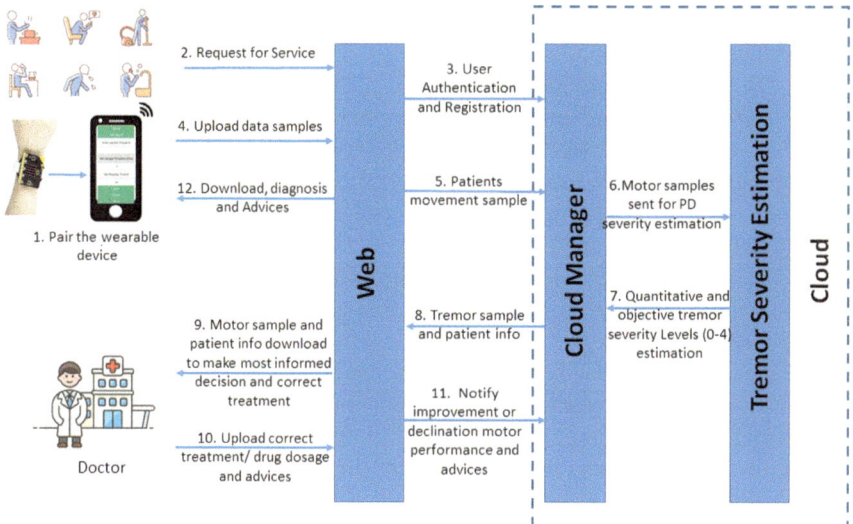

Fig. 5.1   Pipeline of data processing inside cloud

The DL algorithm could either be directly integrated into the platform using JavaScript or executed locally on a computer via a Python or MATLAB script. The algorithm's output can then be relayed back to the platform for further processing.

5.1.2   Cloud-based Parkinson's Disease Severity Estimation Framework

The cloud infrastructure combines both hardware and software components, with the hardware primarily managed by the service provider and the software largely residing on the client side. Within this context, Platform as a Service (PaaS) encompasses aspects such as design, modeling, development, testing, databases, and web servers.

The system's workflow within the cloud structure is illustrated in Fig. 5.1. The sequence of tasks is outlined as follows:

Step 1 Individuals with Parkinson's disease (PwPD) wear the bracelet on their most affected limb, establish a connection between the device and their smartphone, and proceed with Data-Logging Activities (DLAs).

Step 2 The patient utilizing the bracelet initiates a service request to the ServiceNow platform using their smartphone.

Step 3 The patient's identity is authenticated and verified by the cloud manager module, which employs the credentials entered during the cloud login process.

Step 4 Once registered within the cloud, the patient records and uploads motor samples using the bracelet, which remains connected to the mobile app.

Step 5 The accelerometer samples are transmitted via the internet to the cloud manager module.

Step 6 The cloud manager module directs the raw sensor data to the Parkinson's disease (PD) detection system, where the sample is stored and evaluated.

Step 7 The PD detection system processes and scrutinizes the inertial sensor signals from the patient, furnishing quantitative analysis. Subsequently, it transmits the data back to the cloud manager module for further evaluation of severity levels using deep learning (DL).

Step 8 The cloud manager module conveys the analyzed samples, along with patient information, to a web page that is also updated in the mobile app. This data is accessible to doctors for review.

Step 9 Medical professionals download the signal assessment results and patient information to provide treatment recommendations based on the observed motor impairments.

Step 10 Doctors review and upload the diagnosis, including the severity level, and provide guidance via the web interface.

Step 11 The cloud manager module receives these updates via the internet and promptly notifies the patient accordingly.

5.1.3 ServiceNow Platform: Cloud Based Monitoring Platform

First, the ServiceNow platform is used to host the custom A-WEAR UI component which offers a friendly user interface for accessing the A-WEAR bracelet. It offers features such as registering patients, getting new reads from them as shown in Fig. 5.2, and orchestrating the prediction result and training of DL model. With the new user interface (UI) components from ServiceNow, it is possible now to develop a full custom web application with all the features and capabilities that a web application can offer.

The A-WEAR application uses the Core Bluetooth framework in order to leverage the Bluetooth capability of the device that is running on. This means that you can develop the application once, and use it on any kind of device (phone, table, computer) that has a browser. Second, the ServiceNow platform is used to store the readings, as the A-WEAR component will create for any new session a record to hold the generated CSV file. The platform also orchestrates the training of the DL that is hosted on a MID Server (Java agent used for local execution of commands).

As the process above shows, training the DL model can be also triggered directly from the A-WEAR app. After the gathered data is labeled, a new training set record can be created to hold the data in ServiceNow and also gets back the results of the training. The training set unique number has just to be entered and once the progress of the training started, it is logged into the A-WEAR Application interface. Once the training session is started, a custom developed ServiceNow flow triggers the

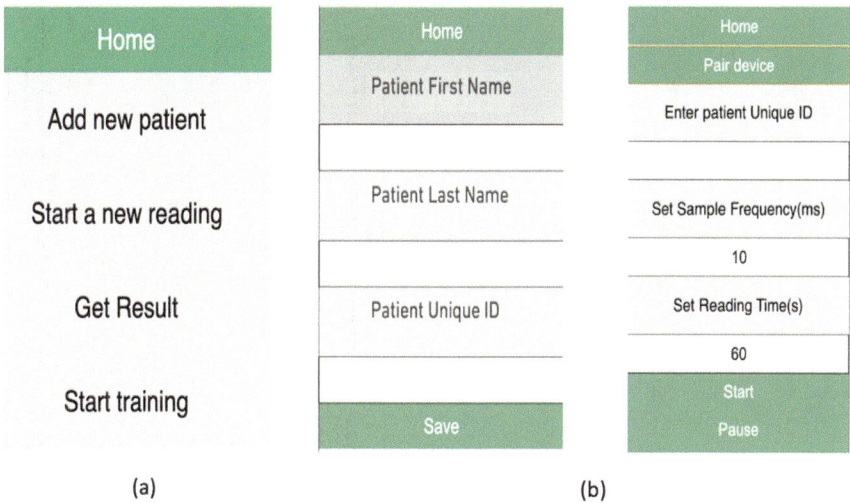

Fig. 5.2 **a** illustrates the main interface of the bespoke ServiceNow UI Component, while **b** portrays the screen dedicated to patient registration and data retrieval within the custom ServiceNow UI Component

execution of the python scripts in charge of training the deep learning network by using the MID Server Java agent that runs on a local server. Once all three major steps of the training are executed, the updated neural network configuration after the training is saved locally on the MID Server (the server where the MID agent is installed). Figures 5.3 and 5.4 show front-end and back-end structure of the platform.

The training trials were conducted on a Supermicro server equipped with two Intel(R) Xeon(R) CPU X5690 processors, each operating at 3.47 GHz. The server boasts a cumulative count of 24 logical cores and approximately 30 GB of RAM. It operates on a Debian distribution.

The employed datasets, averaging around 10–11 MB, were subjected to timing measurements for each execution step. These timings were recorded from the commencement of the training session within the A-WEAR application until the final outcomes were uploaded to the ServiceNow platform. The average execution time for each step is outlined in Table 5.1.

Here * the execution time also includes retrieval of CSV dataset file from ServiceNow platform (for filter step) and upload of output training graphs back to the ServiceNow platform (classification step)—the retrieval and upload operation are performed via REST API and ** the total time also includes the ServiceNow platform specific operation regarding database read and update.

During the execution of a single training session, the maximum reported CPU usage percentage was around 27% as shown in Fig. 5.6.

During the training session, the utilization of RAM memory remains within the normal range observed by the Debian operating system (approximately 3 GB), as illustrated in Fig. 5.7.

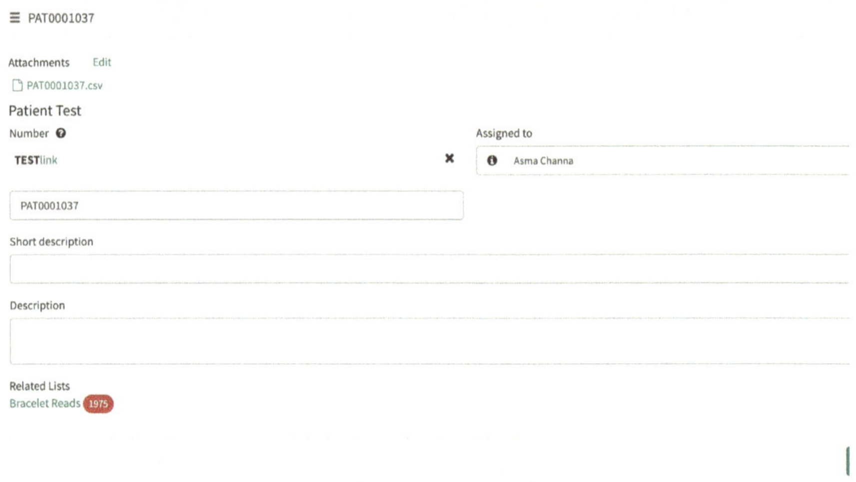

☰ PAT0001037

Attachments   Edit
🗋 PAT0001037.csv
Patient Test
Number ❓   Assigned to
TESTlink   ✖   ❶ Asma Channa

PAT0001037

Short description

Description

Related Lists
Bracelet Reads 1975

Fig. 5.3 The patient data retrieval interface on the front-end portal page presents the A-WEAR readings captured during a single session. This includes both individual readings and a CSV file representation

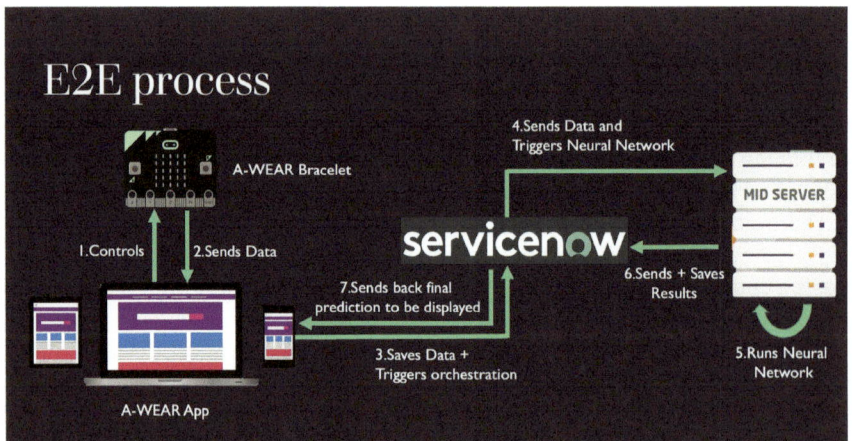

Fig. 5.4 The comprehensive process flow spanning the A-WEAR Bracelet (controlled by the micro:bit controller), the A-WEAR Application (integrated ServiceNow UI Component), and the MID Server responsible for executing the DL operations

Upon the initiation of a new training session, the MID Server, responsible for conducting the training, initially retrieves the CSV dataset associated with the chosen session from the ServiceNow platform. The average response time for obtaining a dataset of approximately 10–11 MB through REST API registers around 7410 ms, contributing to the overall execution time noted in Table 5.1.

Table 5.1 Mean execution times for datasets of size 10–11 MB

Class (Training steps)	Execution time (ms)
Filter	14338*
Feature extraction	6408
Classification	26573*
Total time	49011**

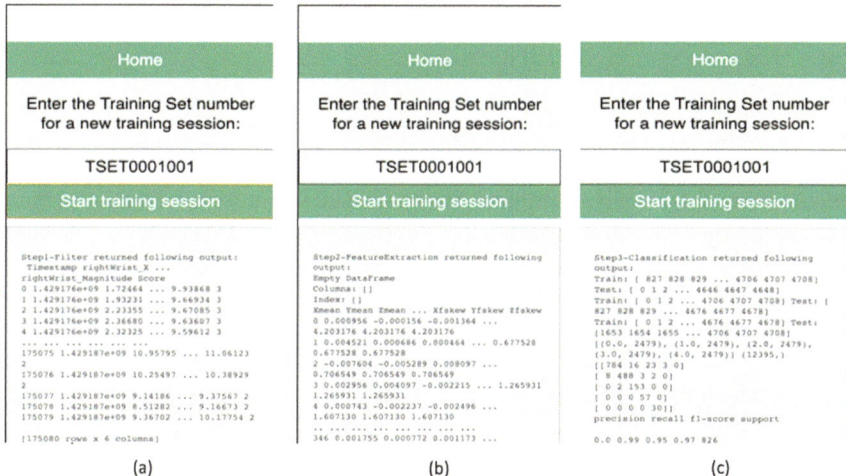

(a)   (b)   (c)

Fig. 5.5 Training Session application screen (**a**) shows Filter Step of training executed and logged into the application, (**b**) shows Feature Extraction Step of training executed and logged into the application and (**c**) depicts Classification Step of training executed and logged into the application

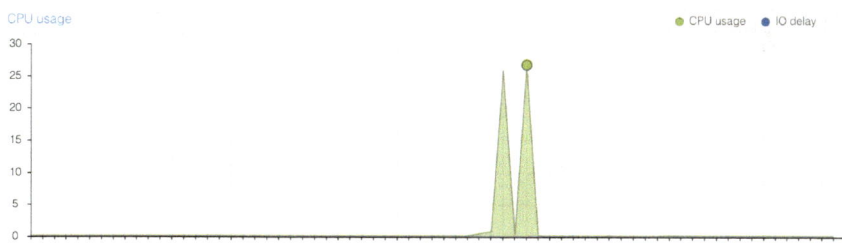

Fig. 5.6 CPU usage percentage usage during two consecutive training session—the green spikes represent the training sessions

Throughout the training session, the A-WEAR mobile app queries the output logs from each step, which are logged in the ServiceNow platform, every 5 s. This real-time querying, aimed at displaying the latest training progress to the user (as depicted in Fig. 5.5), incurs a response time of about 10–12 ms. Importantly, these queries have no discernible impact on the total execution time of the training session.

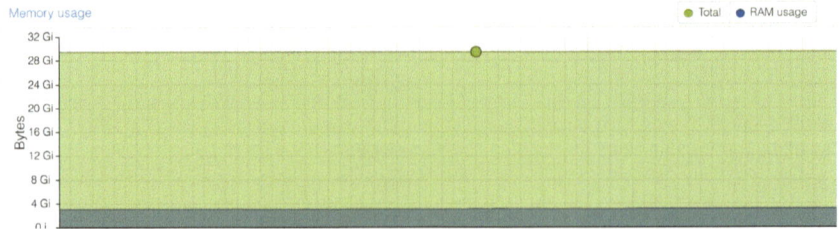

Fig. 5.7 RAM usage remains constant during two consecutive training sessions

At the conclusion of the training session, the resultant output graphs are transmitted back to the ServiceNow platform through REST API. These graphs collectively amount to around 105 KB of data, with an upload response time of approximately 965 ms. Notably, this response time is encompassed within the total execution time detailed in Table 5.1. It's noteworthy that this time is based on the premise that three distinct output graphs exist for each training session, and each PNG file is uploaded individually through a separate REST call.

In conclusion, employing the ServiceNow platform's latest features enables training sessions for datasets comprising 10–11 MB of data to be executed within a minute or less, with minimal strain on the operational server.

Chapter 6
Predicting Wearing-Off Episodes in Parkinson's with Multimodal Machine Learning

Abstract This chapter addresses the significant concern of wearing-off episodes in patients with Parkinson. These episodes occur when the effects of medication, like levodopa, wear off, resulting in the recurrence of PD symptoms. The methodology harnesses features derived from heart rate, stress levels, sleep patterns, and step counts, combined with machine learning techniques, to forecast wearing-off in patients. Relevant features encompass mean condition, sleep-related factors, and time-related aspects. The study conducts experiments employing five different machine learning algorithms for all participants, seeking a personalized approach. Among the classifiers tested, the XGBoost classifier excels, achieving a 0.43 F1-score and 0.72 balanced accuracy. This methodology presents a promising avenue for automated, sensor-based detection of medication wearing off in PD patients, offering valuable insights into timely intervention and enhanced management strategies.

6.1 Understanding Wearing-Off State in Parkinson's Disease Patients

The management of Parkinson's disease (PD) patients necessitates a multifaceted approach, encompassing lifestyle modifications, therapy, and medication. Patients are often recommended to engage in exercises or various therapies (such as physical, occupational, or speech therapy) as these activities have been demonstrated to ameliorate symptoms [1]. Medications also play a pivotal role in symptom management for PD. One of the primary medications prescribed to PD patients is levodopa, which the brain utilizes to produce dopamine. Elevated dopamine levels help mitigate PD symptoms. Since patients might experience a recurrence of PD symptoms when the medication's effects diminish, it's crucial for patients to take their next dose preemptively. Recognizing the potential for improved quality of life for PD patients through the automated detection of PD symptoms and the wearing-off of medications, researchers have increasingly focused on this area [2].

In this context, the present study elaborates on an approach for the automated identification of medication wearing-off in PD patients using data from the 5th ABC

Challenge Wearing-off Recognition competition. The challenge dataset encompasses measurements from twelve PD patients, monitoring heart rate, stress levels, sleep patterns, and step counts over periods lasting between 7 and 9 days. Patients are also required to self-report drug intake times and the emergence of wearing-off symptoms. For each participant, the challenge mandates participating teams to predict the occurrence of wearing-off 15 min into the future.

Research efforts aimed at identifying wearing-off in PD patients have been continuous in the field. For instance, in a study by Farzanehfar et al. [3], objective determination of wearing-off is pursued. The authors investigated 200 patients, utilizing Parkinson's KinetiGraph (PKG) measurements alongside clinician assessments and quality of life scores to detect the presence of wearing-off. Over the span of one month, patients received incremental adjustments to their therapy while continuously wearing the PKG logger. Comparisons were made between measurements taken at the beginning and the end of the month, revealing that 43% of patients exhibited wearing-off, leading to therapy adjustments. This study underscored the value of objective measurements in detecting wearing-off. In a more recent work by Farzanehfar et al. [4], a comparison was drawn between conventional PD patient care and a care approach based on sensor-acquired data. The study employed sensors to measure bradykinesia scores in patients, conducting controlled trials across different groups.

In the study conducted by Victorino et al. [5], an exploration of the relationship between levodopa drug wearing-off in Parkinson's patients and fitness tracker data is presented. The authors gathered data from a 30-day period involving two patients. The fitness tracker collected metrics such as heart rate, stress (assessed via Electrodermal Activity—EDA), step count, and sleep patterns. Additionally, patients were required to provide information about their drug intake, instances of wearing-off, and a range of impairments, which were evaluated using the Wearing-Off Questionnaire (WoQ-9) [6] to assess their quality of life.

The analysis conducted by the authors revealed a significant correlation between the time elapsed since the last medication intake and the occurrence of wearing-off symptoms. Moreover, step count and sleep duration emerged as potential predictors of the wearing-off state. Building upon their prior work, the authors proposed a multimodal detection scheme for Parkinson's wearing-off in a subsequent study [7]. Feature extraction encompassed computations of various sleep stage durations, their proportions, and sleep efficiency. The collected data was then aggregated, and five distinct machine learning algorithms—logistic regression (LR), linear support vector machine (LSVM), decision tree (DT), random forest (RFC), and gradient boosting (GB)—were evaluated individually for each patient. Notably, the authors achieved balanced accuracy exceeding 70% for every participant.

It's worth highlighting that the authors of this research favored the development of personalized models, rather than relying on a generalized model applicable to all subjects.

The primary innovation of this study lies in the formulation of statistically robust biomarkers for detecting wearing-off states in Parkinson's disease (PD) patients. Furthermore, a noteworthy accomplishment of this research is the development of a machine learning model using XGBoost, achieving a substantial F1-score of 0.43 and a balanced accuracy of 0.72 for forecasting the wearing-off state. Additionally, the study explores personalized prediction models. Another significant contribution is the provision of model interpretability, which has enabled the identification of valuable features including those related to sleep, mean condition, and time.

6.2 Methodology

Here we first describe the dataset and then discuss the conducted experiment.

6.2.1 Dataset

The dataset utilized in this study was sourced from the 5th ABC Challenge—Wearing-Off Recognition [8]. The data was captured through Garmin fitness trackers, providing records encompassing sleep stages (light, deep, REM, awake) and their respective durations, stress levels, heart rates, and step counts. Heart rate intervals were at 15 s increments, stress scores at 3 min intervals, and step counts at 15 min intervals. Additionally, the dataset included information about drug intake linked with concurrent wearing-off symptoms, as well as distinct details regarding instances of wearing-off periods and the associated encountered symptoms. These details were collected from patients using the Wearing-Off Questionnaire (WoQ-9) [7], with symptoms encompassing pain, tremors, anxiety, rigidity, slowdown, slow thoughts, impaired hands, mood changes, and muscle spasms. The challenge organizers provided both a 10-person training dataset, a 2-person training dataset, and a 10-person testing dataset.

Following resampling and labeling, 379 wearing-off and 4269 non-wearing-off samples were included in the 10-person dataset, along with 94 wearing-off and 556 non-wearing-off samples in the 2-person dataset. The labeling methodology aligned with the organizers' guidelines [8]. Additionally, a challenge test dataset comprised 1798 samples, each spanning 15 min.

Furthermore, participant information was available for the 10-person dataset, comprising 7 women and 3 men. The mean age for women was 50.13 ± 8.64, while for men, it was 73.00 ± 10.99. Other metrics assessing Parkinson's disease (PD) were as follows for women: Hoehn and Yahr scale 2.5 ± 0.5, Japan Ministry of Health, Labor, and Welfare's classification of living dysfunction (JCLD) 1.63 ± 0.49, and PD Questionnaire (PDQ-8) $44.14\% \pm 17.29\%$. Correspondingly, for men, the metrics were as follows: Hoehn and Yahr scale of 3.33 ± 0.47, JCLD 2.0 ± 0.0, and PDQ-8 $39.58\% \pm 14.51$.

6.2.2   Experiment Description

The algorithm's workflow is depicted in Fig. 6.1. To begin, the dataset underwent resampling to consolidate all modalities, selecting a 15 min time window as the outcome of this process. Feature extraction predominantly occurred concurrently with the resampling step. Features computed during resampling included mean, standard deviation (std), maximum (max), minimum (min), range, approximate entropy, Shannon entropy, skew, slope, kurtosis, residual standard deviation (rsd), variance, and weighted averages for steps, sleep, heart rate, and the number of steps taken. Additional sleep-related features comprised the sum of deep and light stages (nonrem_total), the sum of deep, light, and REM stages (total), non-REM percentage (ratio of nonrem_total to total multiplied by 100%), and sleep efficiency (ratio of total to the sum of total and awake stages).

Furthermore, features were extracted from the pycatch22 library [9], and cyclic time features recommended by challenge organizers—time of day, day of the week, and hour features—were added. Activity features, expressed as ratios of heart rate-related to corresponding step features, were computed, along with efficiency features (ratios of stress-related to step-related features) and condition features (ratios of stress-related to heart rate-related features). For instance, activity_mean represented the ratio of mean heart rate to mean step count. Inspiration for these features was drawn from reference [10].

Statistical evaluation was performed on all extracted features. The Shapiro-Wilk test determined normal distribution for each group's samples. The two-tailed t-test with $\alpha = 0.05$ significance level was applied, and false discovery rate (FDR) correction was computed to mitigate type I error influence.

For training data labeling, drug intake and the subsequent 15 min were considered. Registered symptoms indicated a wearing-off period during that time. Patient-registered wearing-off periods provided the second source of labeling. Resampled samples within those periods were labeled. The data were then transformed into a supervised format, containing information from two previous samples and labels of the next sample forecasting wearing-off occurrence in the next 15 min.

Next, minimum redundancy maximum relevance algorithm (mRMR) was employed for feature pre-selection, selecting the top 50 features. Hyperparameter tuning followed, and the classification step employed 10-fold cross-validation, including standardization and optional Synthetic Minority Oversampling Technique (SMOTE) augmentation [11]. Utilized classifiers encompassed XGBoost, k-Nearest Neighbors (kNN), Logistic Regression, Decision Tree, and Random Forest. Forecasting outcomes were obtained, and finally, the SHapley Additive exPlanations (SHAP) values provided interpretability for the XGBoost model.

Calculation of SHAP values applied to XGBoost predictions utilizing a dataset comprising twelve individuals.

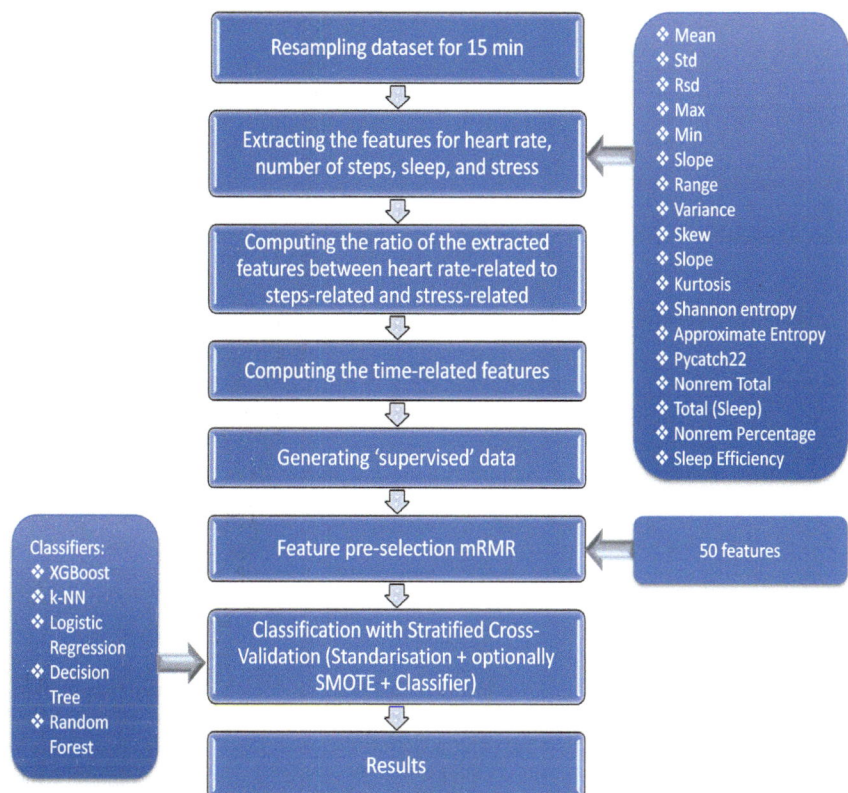

Fig. 6.1 Methodology

6.3   Results and Discussion

The two-tailed t-test was conducted on a dataset of 12 individuals. The data's normality was met for the analyzed features. Following the application of the Benjamini-Hochberg procedure to control type I error, a total of 158 features out of 340 were identified. The 30 most successful features that passed the test are detailed in Table 6.1. Notably, cyclic hour-related features emerged as some of the most significant markers, including timestamp_hour_cos(t), timestamp_hour_cos(t–1), and timestamp_hour_cos(t–2). Subsequently, a set of sleep-related features demonstrated significance, with notable ones being sleep_efficiency(t), total(t), nonrem_percentage(t), nonrem_total(t), sleep_efficiency(t–1), and total(t–1).

Furthermore, several features extracted through the pycatch22 library garnered attention. In addition, specific stress-related features proved valuable: stress_max(t) and (t–1), stress_weighted_average(t) and (t–1), and stress_mean(t) and (t–1). Additionally, condition_weighted_average(t) and condition_weighted_average(t–1) were identified as valuable features. These features represent the ratio of mean heart rate

Table 6.1 Two-tailed t-test including also FDR correction for the wearing-off and non-wearing off groups for 12-person dataset

Feature	pval	pval_FDR	Feature	pval	pval_FDR
timestamp_hour_cos(t)	4.69E–22	1.59E–19	hr_FC_LocalSimple _mean3_stderr(t)	4.77E–13	1.01E–11
sleep_efficiency(t)	1.15E–21	1.96E–19	stress_max(t)	6.37E–12	1.27E–10
timestamp_hour_cos(t–1)	2.41E–21	2.05E–19	nonrem_total(t–2)	7.12E–12	1.35E–10
total(t)	2.21E–21	2.05E–19	light(t–1)	1.80E–11	3.23E–10
nonrem_percentage(t)	5.00E–21	3.40E–19	hr_SP_Summaries _welch_rect_centroid(t)	2.65E–11	4.50E–10
timestamp_hour_cos(t–2)	1.75E–20	9.94E–19	hr_MD_hrv_classic_pnn40(t)	3.83E–11	6.20E–10
nonrem_total(t)	1.88E–19	9.14E–18	stress_weighted_average(t)	7.83E–11	1.21E–09
sleep_efficiency(t–1)	4.32E–18	1.84E–16	stress_mean(t)	1.22E–10	1.73E–09
total(t–1)	1.01E–17	3.82E–16	condition_weighted_average(t)	1.22E–10	1.73E–09
nonrem_percentage(t–1)	3.82E–17	1.30E–15	stress_weighted _average(t–1)	1.40E–10	1.91E–09
nonrem_total(t–1)	3.11E–15	9.61E–14	stress_max(t–1)	1.60E–10	2.10E–09
light(t)	6.69E–15	1.90E–13	stress_mean(t–1)	1.75E–10	2.13E–09
sleep_efficiency(t–2)	1.42E–14	3.71E–13	hr_SB_TransitionMatrix _3ac_sumdiagcov(t)	1.76E-10	2.13E–09
total(t–2)	3.19E–14	7.74E–13	hr_SB_BinaryStats_diff _longstretch0(t)	6.21E–10	7.28E–09
nonrem_percentage(t–2)	1.27E–13	2.87E–12	condition_weighted_average(t–1)	4.26E–09	4.83E–08

to the mean number of steps taken during the analyzed time window and a 15 min sample from before.

The most favorable results for predicting wearing-off states in the dataset of 12 participants were achieved using the XGBoost classifier (refer to Table 6.2). The highest F1-score (0.43), balanced accuracy (0.72), and MCC (0.37) were recorded. Conversely, Logistic Regression yielded poor results, with an F1-score of 0.01.

Furthermore, Fig. 6.2 illustrates the interpretability of the general XGBoost model. The most significant and positively correlated feature linked to the wearing-off state was found to be condition_weighted_average(t). This indicates that during the wearing-off symptoms, individuals might experience a worsened physical condition due to exertion. A longer duration of light sleep during the night was associated with a higher likelihood of detecting the wearing-off state, positively correlating with this feature. Conversely, timestamp_hour_cos(t) and timestamp_hour_cos(t–2) showed negative correlations with the wearing-off state, while timestamp_hour_sin(t–2) displayed a positive correlation. Notably, when sleep_efficiency(t) is lower, indicating potential sleep disruption, there is a heightened probability of the wearing-off state being detected.

The study introduced an automated methodology for detecting wearing-off states. Literature has recognized heart rate, stress levels, and sleep patterns as valuable predictors of Parkinson's disease [7], justifying the use of fitness trackers for predicting wearing-off states. About half of the proposed features were statistically significant, with those related to sleep, stress, mean condition, and time showing particular importance. XGBoost emerged as the most suitable classifier for forecasting wearing-off

Table 6.2 The classification outcomes for the dataset comprising 12 participants

Classifier	SMOTE	F1-score	Balanced accuracy	Sensitivity	Specificity	MCC	Recall	Precision
XGBoost	–	**0.43 (0.05)**	**0.72 (0.03)**	0.54 (0.07)	0.91 (0.01)	**0.37 (0.05)**	0.54 (0.07)	0.37 (0.04)
XGBoost	+	0.39 (0.06)	0.64 (0.03)	0.31 (0.06)	**0.97 (0.01)**	0.36 (0.07)	0.31 (0.06)	**0.52 (0.08)**
k-NN	–	0.37 (0.07)	0.63 (0.03)	0.29 (0.07)	0.97 (0.01)	0.34 (0.07)	0.29 (0.07)	0.51 (0.09)
k-NN	+	0.36 (0.05)	0.66 (0.03)	0.41(0.07)	0.91 (0.01)	0.29 (0.06)	0.41 (0.07)	0.32 (0.05)
Logistic regression	–	0.01 (0.02)	0.50 (0.00)	0.00 (0.01)	1.00 (0.00)	0.01 (0.05)	0.00 (0.01)	0.13 (0.31)
Logistic regression	+	0.25 (0.02)	0.65 (0.03)	**0.66 (0.07)**	0.64 (0.02)	0.17 (0.04)	**0.66 (0.07)**	0.15 (0.01)
Decision tree	–	0.23 (0.02)	0.63 (0.03)	0.65 (0.06)	0.61 (0.03)	0.15 (0.04)	0.65 (0.06)	0.14 (0.01)
Decision tree	+	0.23 (0.02)	0.63 (0.03)	0.65 (0.06)	0.61 (0.03)	0.15 (0.04)	0.65 (0.06)	0.14 (0.01)
Random forest	–	0.26 (0.03)	0.66 (0.04)	0.63 (0.10)	0.68 (0.04)	0.19 (0.05)	0.63 (0.10)	0.17 (0.02)
Random forest	+	0.24 (0.03)	0.62 (0.04)	0.59 (0.14)	0.65 (0.13)	0.15 (0.05)	0.59 (0.14)	0.15 (0.03)

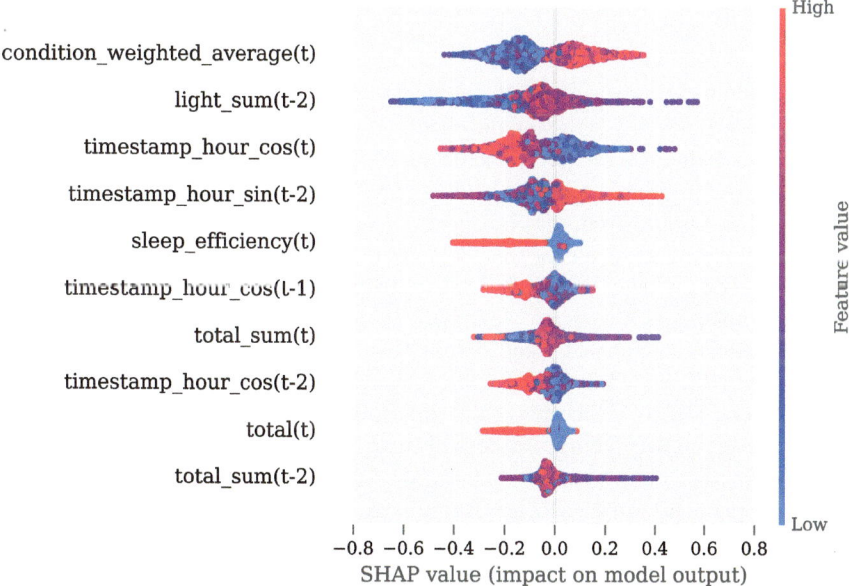

Fig. 6.2 Calculation of SHAP values applied to XGBoost predictions utilizing a dataset comprising twelve individuals

Table 6.3 The outcomes of the classification for models pertaining to 10 individual patients

Participant	F1-score	Balanced accuracy	Sensitivity	Specificity	MCC	Recall	Precision	Wearing-off	Nr. samples
1	0.29 (0.26)	0.64 (0.15)	0.33 (0.29)	0.96 (0.03)	0.27 (0.27)	0.33 (0.29)	0.29 (0.30)	25	505
2	0.00 (0.00)	**0.83 (0.22)**	0.00 (0.00)	**1.00 (0.00)**	0.00 (0.02)	0.00 (0.00)	0.00 (0.00)	3	115
3	0.56 (0.14)	0.75 (0.08)	0.55 (0.17)	0.95 (0.03)	0.51 (0.15)	0.55 (0.17)	0.60 (0.15)	85	691
4	0.58 (0.16)	0.74 (0.09)	0.52 (0.18)	0.97 (0.02)	0.55 (0.17)	0.52 (0.18)	0.69 (0.18)	76	698
5	0.12 (0.25)	0.55 (0.12)	0.12 (0.24)	0.98 (0.02)	0.10 (0.27)	0.12 (0.24)	0.14 (0.31)	20	397
6	0.43 (0.19)	0.71 (0.12)	0.50 (0.24)	0.92 (0.04)	0.38 (0.21)	0.50 (0.24)	0.39 (0.19)	43	510
7	0.00 (0.00)	1.00 (0.00)	0.00 (0.00)	**1.00 (0.00)**	0.00 (0.00)	0.00 (0.00)	0.00 (0.00)	0	31
8	0.47 (0.25)	0.69 (0.12)	0.39 (0.24)	0.99 (0.02)	0.48 (0.26)	0.39 (0.24)	0.67 (0.34)	40	604
9	0.55 (0.22)	0.80 (0.14)	0.64 (0.27)	0.95 (0.03)	0.53 (0.23)	0.64 (0.27)	0.52 (0.25)	34	499
10	**0.67 (0.18)**	0.81 (0.11)	**0.65 (0.22)**	0.98 (0.02)	**0.66 (0.19)**	**0.65 (0.22)**	**0.75 (0.20)**	53	610

states among those tested, although augmentation did not enhance its performance. Interestingly, Logistic Regression did succeed with augmentation.

However, individual models to predict wearing-off states for 10 participants were less successful in 4 cases compared to the model developed for the larger 12-person dataset. SHAP values from the XGBoost model affirmed the significance of mean condition, time-related features, and sleep-related biomarkers.

This study does have limitations, such as missing values due to participants occasionally forgetting to wear the wearable [7]. Additionally, the feature-extraction dataset includes aggregated sleep records and information from earlier samples than the two already analyzed. While combining modalities with gyroscopic and accelerometer signals could increase accuracy, it would demand more accurate and costly devices, making them less accessible for PD patients [7]. Furthermore, personalized models are advantageous in acknowledging the varying symptom experiences among PD patients [5]. Nevertheless, some personalized models in this study yielded less satisfactory results (patient 1, patient 2, patient 5, patient 7; refer to Table 6.3).

6.4 Conclusion

Detecting the decline in medication effectiveness among PD patients is crucial for delivering appropriate care. However, there's a shortage of automated techniques that utilize sensor data to perform such detection. Building upon the 5th ABC challenge on Wearing-off recognition, this research work introduces a method that leverages data from various measurements: stress levels, step counts, heart rate, sleep patterns, and patient information. The aim is to predict instances of medication wearing-off over 15 min intervals for ten patients.

Numerous features were derived from these measured parameters, encompassing basic statistical attributes and more specialized traits such as the catch22 feature set. Among these, the most pertinent features were those related to mean condition, time, and sleep patterns. To forecast wearing-off states, five distinct machine-learning algorithms were tested. This study went beyond the use of individual models, as explored in a relevant paper [7], by also evaluating predictions from a general model.

Results indicated that XGBoost yielded the most favorable performance: achieving an F1-score of 0.43 and a balanced accuracy of 0.72. Looking ahead, potential future endeavors involve predicting medication wearing-off prior to patients themselves being consciously aware, along with expanding the dataset.

References

1. M. Fayyaz, S. S. Jaffery, F. Anwer, A. Zil-E-Ali, and I. Anjum, *The effect of physical activity in Parkinson's disease: a mini-review*, Cureus, vol. 10, no. 7, 2018, Cureus.
2. J. N. Victorino, Y. Shibata, S. Inoue, and T. Shibata, *Forecasting Parkinson's Disease Patients – Wearing-Off using Wrist-Worn Fitness Tracker and Smartphone Dataset*, ABC 2022, 2022.
3. P. Farzanehfar, H. Woodrow, and M. Horne, *Assessment of Wearing Off in Parkinson's disease using objective measurement*, Journal of Neurology, vol. 268, pp. 914–922, 2021, Springer.
4. P. Farzanehfar, H. Woodrow, and M. Horne, *Sensor Measurements Can Characterize Fluctuations and Wearing Off in Parkinson's Disease and Guide Therapy to Improve Motor, Non-motor and Quality of Life Scores*, Frontiers in Aging Neuroscience, vol. 14, p. 852992, 2022, Frontiers.
5. J. N. Victorino, Y. Shibata, S. Inoue, and T. Shibata, *Understanding Wearing-Off Symptoms in Parkinson's Disease Patients using Wrist-Worn Fitness Tracker and a Smartphone*, Procedia Computer Science, vol. 196, pp. 684–691, 2022, Elsevier.
6. A. Antonini, P. Martinez-Martin, R. K. Chaudhuri, M. Merello, R. Hauser, R. Katzenschlager, P. Odin, M. Stacy, F. Stocchi, W. Poewe, and others, *Wearing-off scales in Parkinson's disease: critique and recommendations*, Movement Disorders, vol. 26, no. 12, pp. 2169–2175, 2011, Wiley Online Library.
7. J. N. Victorino, Y. Shibata, S. Inoue, and T. Shibata, *Predicting Wearing-Off of Parkinson's Disease Patients Using a Wrist-Worn Fitness Tracker and a Smartphone: A Case Study*, Applied Sciences, vol. 11, no. 16, p. 7354, 2021, MDPI.
8. *5th ABC Challenge: Forecasting Parkinson's Disease Patients' Wearing-Off Phenomenon Datasets*, https://ieee-dataport.org/competitions/5th-abc-challenge-forecasting-parkinsons-disease-patients-wearing-phenomenon-datasets, [Accessed: 10-07-2023].
9. *pycatch22 - CAnonical Time-series CHaracteristics in python*, https://github.com/DynamicsAndNeuralSystems/pycatch22, [Accessed: 11-07-2023].
10. T. Mishra et al., *Pre-symptomatic detection of COVID-19 from smartwatch data*, Nature biomedical engineering, vol. 4, no. 12, pp. 1208–1220, 2020, Nature Publishing Group UK London.
11. *SMOTE library*, https://imbalanced-learn.org/stable/references/generated/imblearn.over_sampling.SMOTE.html, [Accessed: 11-07-2023].

Chapter 7
Enhancing Gait Analysis Through Wearable Insoles and Deep Learning Techniques

Abstract This study explores the utilization of wearable sensor insoles for gait signal analysis across diverse participant groups, including elderly individuals, adults, and PD patients. The investigation seeks to establish a connection between changes in stride variability, neurological functionality, and the influence of aging on the human body. To validate the study's findings, participants' gait cycles undergo comparison using the Detrended Fluctuation Analysis (DFA) method, which assesses fluctuations in stride time. The results underscore that stride time fluctuations are more pronounced in elderly subjects and PD patients, implying potential irregularities in the fractal characteristics of lower limb dynamics linked to central nervous system control. Another aspect introduced in this chapter outlines an innovative approach to gait assessment, employing the continuous wavelet transform method. This approach addresses the analysis of idiopathic PD severity levels as well as gait variability in age-matched individuals.

7.1 Overview

Gait cycle variability has significant implications for quality of life (QoL) [1]. In elderly individuals, frequent presence of stride interval variability is considered the fifth leading cause of mortality [2]. Similarly, increased gait alteration in the form of stride interval among PD patients leads to a high risk of falls, with around 50% of PD patients experiencing multiple falls annually [3]. Healthy adults typically exhibit small gait variability, approximately 2% around the mean, but this variability significantly increases in patients with Parkinson's and Huntington's diseases [4]. Despite extensive efforts to comprehend the pathophysiology of falls in elderly individuals and develop preventive measures, addressing the challenging syndrome of gait disability, especially when comparing elderly individuals to those with neurocognitive disorders like PD, remains a significant gap.

7.2 Correlation Between Ageing, Neurological Functioning, and the Variability of Stride Rate and Altered Fractal Dynamics

The process of aging is linked with a decrease in balance, diminished postural stability, and discomfort experienced while standing for prolonged periods. This situation contributes to falls and functional limitations among the elderly. Over the past decade, significant advancements have been made by researchers in this domain. They have put forth wearable devices and artificial intelligence algorithms aimed at detecting falls, assessing the risk of falling, and issuing emergency alerts in the aftermath of a fall [5–7]. These solutions rely on features in the temporal and spatial domains, such as maximum amplitude, minimum amplitude, mean amplitude, variance, kurtosis, and skewness of the signal.

Furthermore, numerous research endeavors [8–10] have concentrated on statistical methods to classify gait patterns related to Parkinson's disease (PD) or extract inherent features. These features encompass an array of temporal and spatial domain parameters. Linear and non-linear functions are utilized to facilitate early PD diagnosis or distinguish between individuals with PD and those who are healthy. However, many of these studies often disregard certain less apparent dynamics and depict the remaining patterns using basic statistical descriptors like averages, mean values, standard deviations, or medians. This approach persists despite the fact that physiological signals frequently exhibit fractal behavior.

Overall, advancements in understanding gait cycle variability and its impact on different populations have led to innovative solutions for fall prevention and diagnosis of NCDs like PD. Yet, there remains a need to explore more sophisticated approaches that consider the complexity and fractal nature of physiological signals, promising a deeper comprehension of gait patterns and enhanced diagnostic capabilities. In this research, we utilized the Detrended Fluctuation Analysis (DFA) algorithm, which characterizes scale-dependent variations known as fluctuations. DFA helps identify fractal scaling properties and long-range correlations in time-dependent signals with discontinuities. Subsequently, we employed the Optimize Support Vector Machine (OSVM) classification method to identify and classify young healthy subjects, elderly adults, and PD patients.

The study aims to achieve two primary objectives:

Investigate potential significant correlations among the three participant groups.

1. Evaluate the conditions under which such correlations exist.
2. Employ the OSVM classifier to distinguish and classify all participants into the respective cohorts of young healthy individuals, elderly adults, and PD patients.

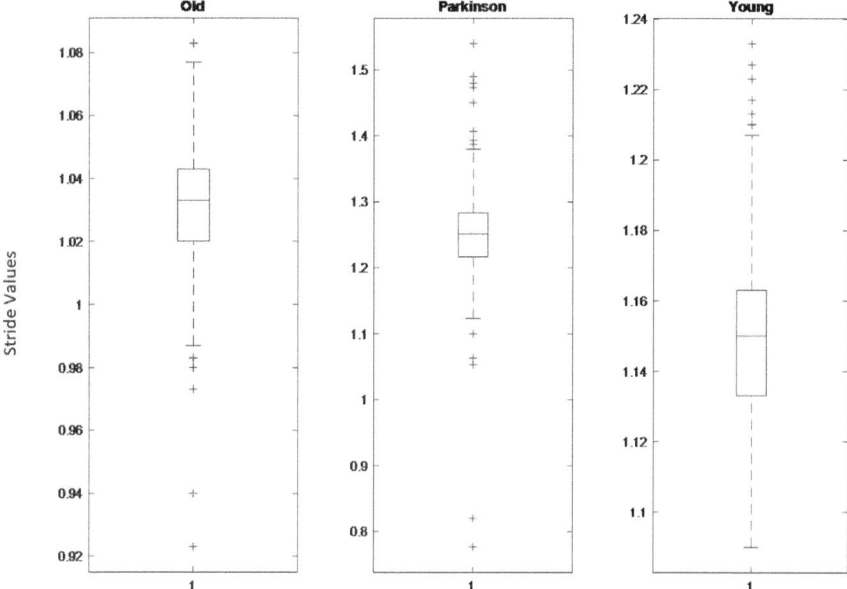

Fig. 7.1 Group comparison of variability of stride time between different groups of subjects

7.3 Methods

7.3.1 Subjects

In this study, we have collected walking stride interval data as time series from a total of 15 participants. The dataset is available in [11]. Among the 15 subjects, 5 have Parkinson's disease (PD) with an average age of 70.4 years and a standard deviation (SD) of 6.406,5 are healthy older adults with an average age of 74.6 years and an SD of 2.05, and the remaining 5 are young participants without any disease, with an average age of 24.4 years and an SD of 2.8. Each participant's data is recorded in two columns: the first column indicates the time stamp (in seconds), and the second column represents the corresponding stride time. Further details of the participants, including their ages, are presented in Table 7.1.

7.3.2 Data Collection

The process of collecting data involved employing ultra-thin force-sensitive resistors that were positioned within the subjects' footwear. The analog force signals were sampled at a frequency of 300 Hz and subsequently transformed into digital signals through a twelve-bit analog-to-digital converter (ADC). To accommodate data stor-

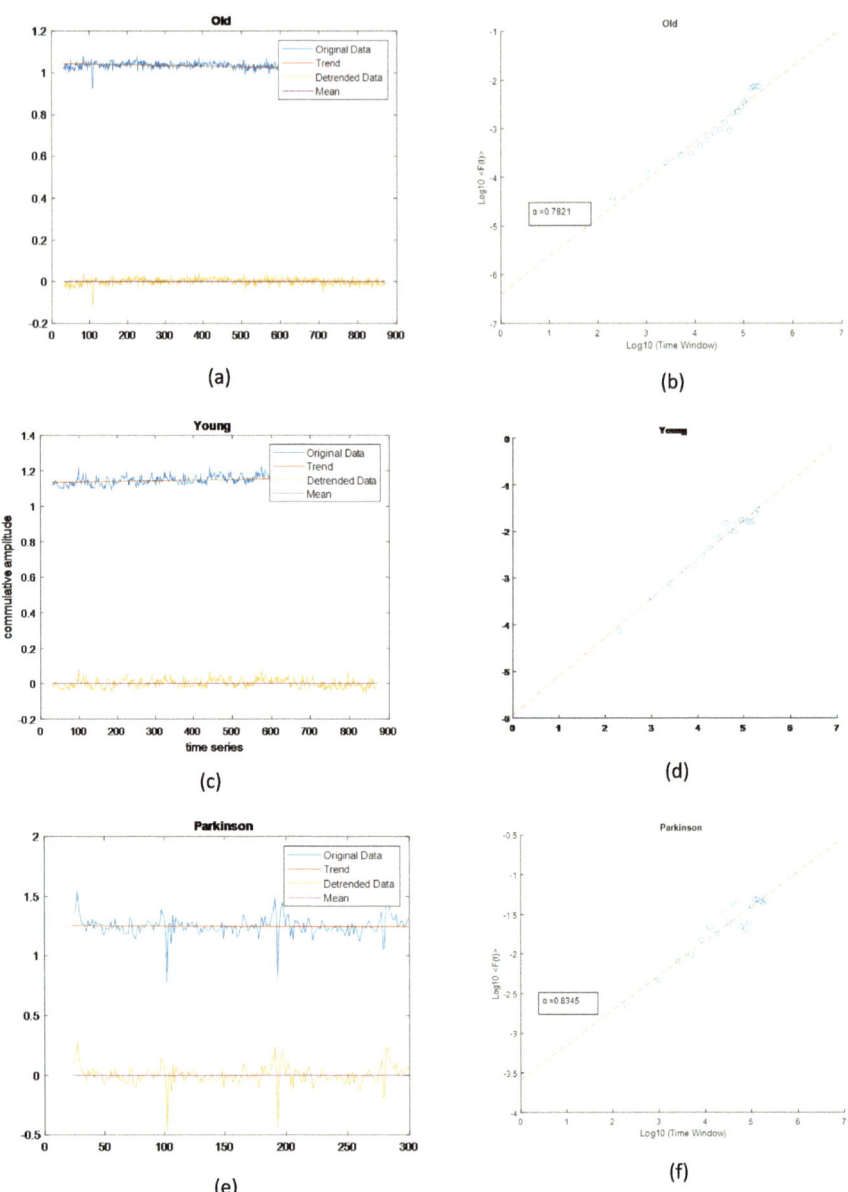

Fig. 7.2 Original time series signal along with the commulative amplitude displaying fluctuations away from the mean i.e., the mean fluctuation per window size on logarithmic axis

Table 7.1 Demographic details of the participants

Patients age	Disease free participants age	
	Old adults	Young adults
60	76	23
66	74	29
75	75	23
74	77	21
77	71	26
Mean ± SD	Mean ± SD	Mean ± SD
70.4 ± 6.4062	74.6 ± 2.05126	24.4 ± 2.8

age requirements, a portable microcomputer was worn around the ankle. This setup enabled the computation of the duration when the foot made contact with the ground.

The data collection procedure comprised two distinct phases. Initially, data was gathered from subjects diagnosed with PD as they engaged in a 6-minute walk, both uphill and downhill within a hallway. Subsequently, data was collected from healthy individuals who walked along roughly circular paths for 15 min. Throughout these trials, all participants maintained a consistent pace on a level surface, navigating an obstacle-free route.

7.3.3 Assessment of Gait Cycle Duration Using DFA

Gait irregularities are observable in both individuals diagnosed with PD and older adults. According to research conducted by [12], fluctuations in stride intervals display fractal dynamics and demonstrate long-range correlations in young and healthy individuals without neurological conditions. In the context of this study, our aim was to explore alterations in the gait cycle that are linked to variations in neurological functioning among adults and the impact of aging. We employed the Detrended Fluctuation Analysis (DFA) technique for this investigation.

DFA is a methodology that identifies elements of long-range correlation and scaling in non-stationary signals. Its non-parametric nature is valuable in preventing the inadvertent identification of apparent long-range correlations that could arise due to nonstationarity.

The DFA method is divided into two parts as in Eqs. 7.1 and 7.2, as demonstrated in the work by [13].

1. the data series $B(k)$ is shifted by the mean and integrated (cumulatively summed),

$$x(k) = \sum_{i=1}^{k}[B(i) - \langle B \rangle] \tag{7.1}$$

Table 7.2 Demographic details of participants

Subjects group	Coefficient α	Fluctuations corresponding to window	Mean absolute error
Old	0.7821	−6.4026	Mean absolute difference between old and PD subjects = 44%
Parkinson	0.4374	−3.5858	Mean absolute difference between PD subjects and young controls = 47%
Young	0.8345	−5.9349	Mean absolute difference between young and old subjects = 6.2%

then it is segmented into a window of $\triangle n$ various sizes. In this way we have illustrated our data profile i.e. $x(k)$. The global trend of the signal is eliminated using subtraction of the mean.

The advantage of utilizing scaling analysis on the signal profile, as opposed to the signal itself, is that it eliminates the need for making assumptions about the signal's stationarity beforehand. By conducting scaling analysis on the signal profile and calculating the scaling exponent (referred to as α), we can estimate the value of H.

2. in each segmentation, the integrated data is locally fit to a polynomial $x_{\triangle n}(k)$ (originally and typically, linear) and the mean-squared residual $F(\triangle n)$ ("fluctuations") is found:

$$F(\triangle n) = \sqrt{1/N \sum_{k-1}^{N}[x(k) - x_{\triangle n}(k)]^2} \tag{7.2}$$

In Eq. 7.2, N represents the total count of data points, while $F^2(\triangle n)$ signifies the mean of the summed squares of the residuals raised within the windows. The nth order polynomial regressor within the DFA framework is commonly designated as DFAn. This procedure investigates self-similarity, which pertains to fractal dynamics, by assessing how the residuals of integrated fluctuations disperse around a regressor at various resolutions (window sizes). If there is a presence of power law scaling, the graph produced by plotting $F(\triangle n)$ against $\triangle n$ in a double logarithmic ("log-log") format, known as the fluctuation plot, generally exhibits a linear relationship.

$$F(\triangle n) = C(\triangle n)^\alpha \Rightarrow ln(F(\triangle n)) = \alpha ln(\triangle n) + ln(C) \tag{7.3}$$

In Eq. 7.3, denoting C as a constant, the scaling exponent α can be estimated through a least-squares fitting process. This scaling exponent α serves as a gauge of correlation within the signal and provides an estimation of the Hurst exponent H. In the context of this study, we employed the DFA method to analyze the stride intervals of various groups: young healthy adults, elderly healthy adults, and patients with Parkinson's disease (PD). This analysis helped assess the correlation present in the gait cycle data. A value of $\alpha = 0.5$ signifies no correlation; if $\alpha < 0.5$, the data displays anticorrelation; and if $\alpha > 0.5$, the data showcases long-range correlation.

7.3.4 Time Series Classification Using Optimizable SVM

Multiple classifiers are utilized for categorizing time series biomedical signals, with the support vector machine (SVM) standing out due to its capability to leverage kernel methods for classification. In our study, we have focused on training the SVM optimally, aiming to achieve effective separation via hyperplanes. However, ensuring high training quality for this classifier depends not solely on the available data but also on additional learning parameters. Regulating these parameters can be complex, especially when dealing with imbalanced datasets.

7.4 Results and Discussion

Wearable sensor data often contain sharp transients and spikes, necessitating pre-processing and visualization before analysis. In the preprocessing step, outliers are removed, and the initial 30 s of data are filtered out to eliminate potential hallway rounds or unwanted noises. Subsequently, the records of the three cohorts are visualized separately and compared using box plots, as illustrated in Fig. 7.1.

The box plot depicted in Fig. 7.1 clearly delineates discernible disparities in median, minimum, and maximum values across each group. To enable accurate fractal analysis of stride interval parameters, the data is subjected to detrending, and the scaling component is computed to illustrate correlations using the DFA methodology. The resultant α values for each group are subsequently utilized for calculating the mean absolute difference, as demonstrated in Table 7.2 and Fig. 7.3.

The application of DFA to ascertain the scaling coefficient characterizes the self-affine nature of the input data. When implementing DFA on non-stationary signals, the objective is to comprehend how the amplitude of oscillation evolves over time. This is achieved by forming a signal profile through cumulative summation of the signal, as defined in Eq. 7.1. A set of window sizes T is established uniformly on a logarithmic scale, based on the signal's length. The signal profile is then divided into distinct time series of length t with 50% overlap, forming the set W. For each window, a least-squares fit is employed to generate a detrended signal, from which the standard deviation is calculated to constitute the fluctuation function as the mean standard

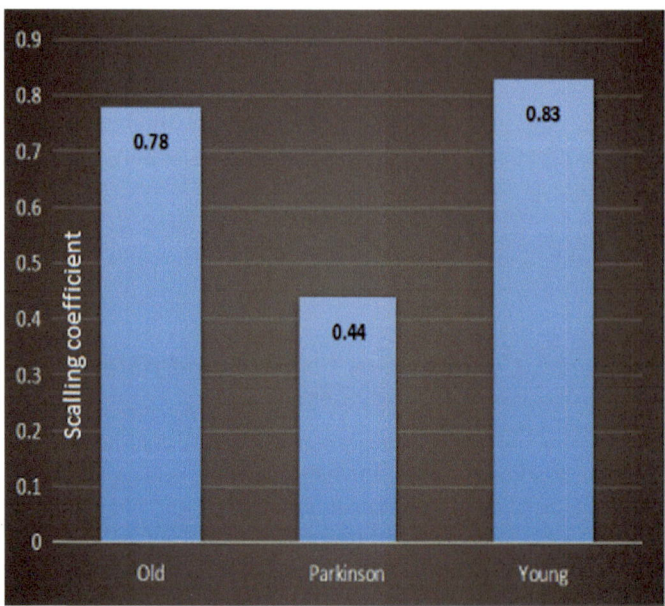

Fig. 7.3 Scaling coefficient of each group

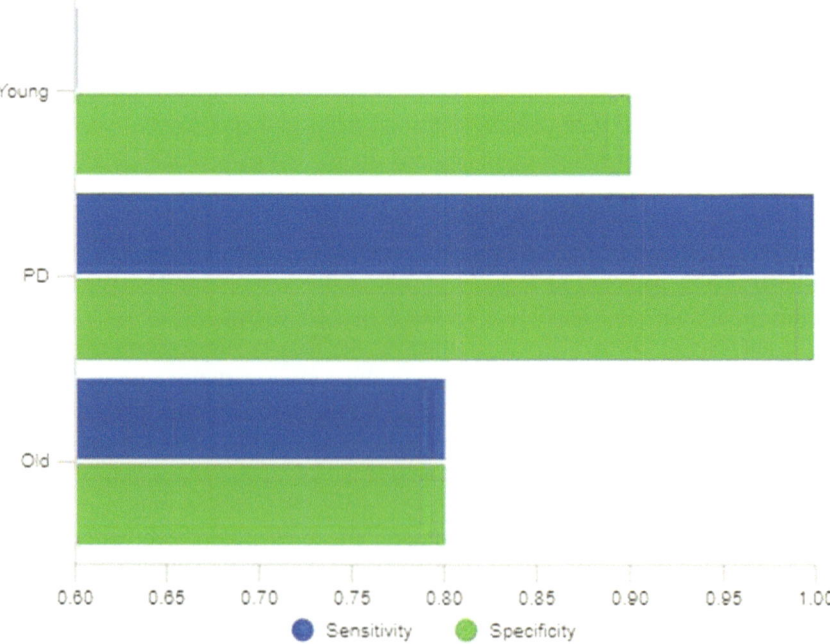

Fig. 7.4 Sensitivity and specificity of each class

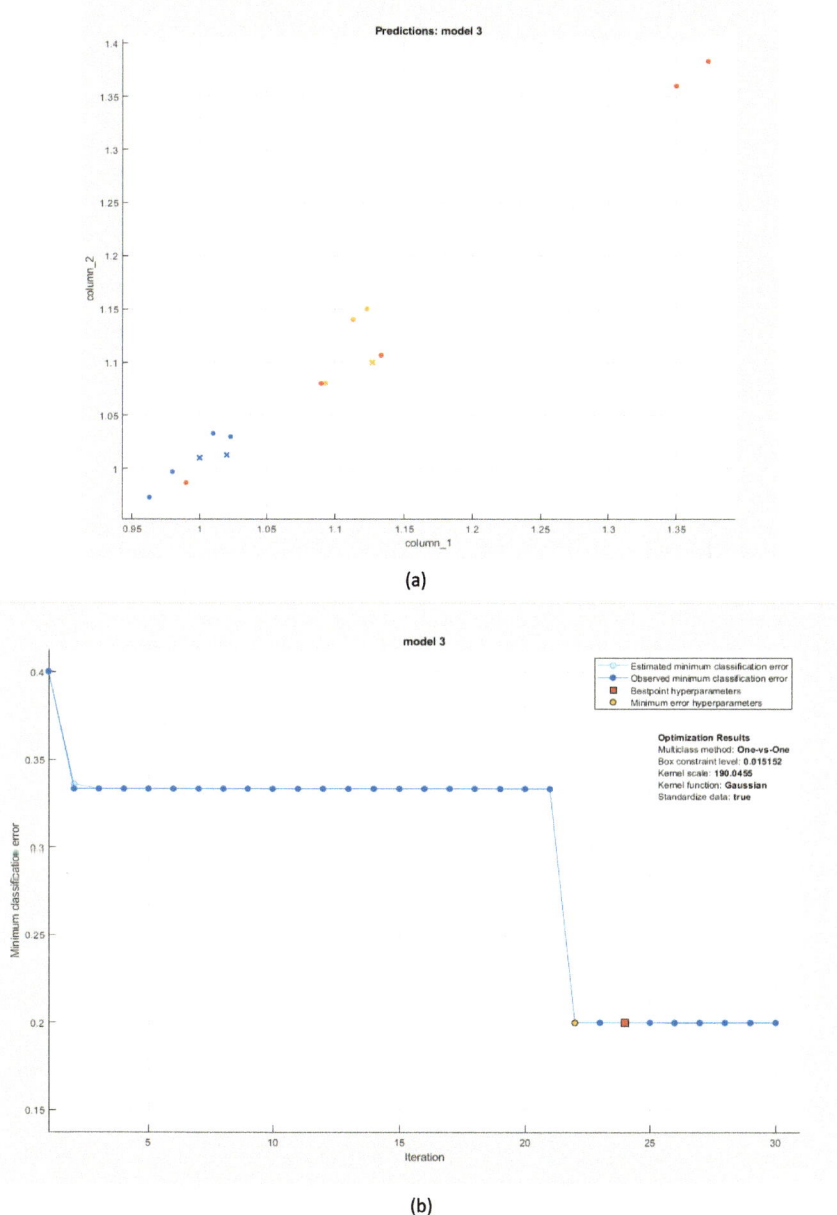

(a)

(b)

Fig. 7.5 a shows model prediction and **b** shows the classification error

deviation of all identically sized windows: $F(t) = \text{mean}(\alpha(W))$. The plots from Fig. 7.2 show the fluctuation function for all window sizes, T, on logarithmic axes and also their DFA fluctuation exponent, α. The fluctuation exponent α is determined as 0.78 for healthy older adults, 0.44 for PD subjects, and 0.68 for healthy young adults. As per [14], an α value below 0.5 for PD patients signifies no correlation, while an α value above 0.5 for healthy subjects denotes long-range correlation. This is vividly illustrated in Fig. 7.3 and Table 7.2.

Automatic classification is carried out on data collected from all three groups, discerning them into three classes through an OSVM classifier. The OSVM classifier effectively selects appropriate input features and optimizes SVM parameters to enhance classification accuracy. Within this study, the OSVM classifier attains an accuracy of 80%. Figure 7.4 visually portrays sensitivity in blue and specificity in green for each group. The PD class demonstrates maximum sensitivity and specificity of 1, contrasting with the healthy young and old cohorts. The young subjects cohort showcases sensitivity of 0.6 and specificity of 0.9, while the older group displays both sensitivity and specificity at 0.8. Figure 7.5a illustrates correct and incorrect predictions, with the cross indicating incorrect predictions and the dot representing correct ones. Notably, the second class exhibits zero incorrect predictions, demonstrating a 100% accuracy rate. Figure 7.5b depicts the reduction of classification error through optimization: from an initial value of 0.4–0.2 post optimization. The yellow circle marks the minimum error value, while the red rectangle signifies the best hyper-parameters point.

This study effectively showcases the appropriateness of employing a fractal approach and the optimizable SVM method for analyzing stride rates in both healthy subjects and a group of PD patients. The research methodology delves into potential correlations among healthy young and old adults and PD patients. Through DFA analysis, it is established that long-range correlation exists between the stride rates of old and young participants (indicated by α values above 0.5), while PD subjects manifest distinct patterns with no similarity. By applying DFA to analyze the gait cycle during short walkways, significant outcomes are obtained, followed by the use of the optimizable SVM classifier to differentiate between these subject cohorts based on their stride intervals. Impressively, the optimizable SVM classifier achieves an accuracy of 80%.

These investigations offer valuable insights into gait irregularities in PD and aging subjects based on their stride cycles, with potential implications for future standardization and incorporation of long-walkways and varied stride intervals in patients with non-communicable diseases (NCDs). This research forms a foundational understanding of gait patterns in PD and aging populations, contributing to advancements in gait analysis techniques and potentially aiding in the diagnosis and management of NCDs.

Table 7.3 The details of dataset participants

Group	No. of recordings	Average age	Age span	Height (cm)	Weight (Kg)	Gender
Parkinson	7	72	63–83	172	81	All males
Adults	13	38	20–58	176	81	11 males, 2 females
Elderly	9	74	60–85	173	80	All males

7.5 Gait Characterization Using Wearable Insoles

Evaluating and managing NCDs requires a thorough assessment of gait patterns. Misunderstandings have arisen due to age-related alterations in gait events, leading to misconceptions when correlating gait variability with NCDs. Precise analysis of gait events is of utmost importance. Common methods such as temporal and spectral feature extraction in gait analysis often overlook critical aspects. Additionally, effectively monitoring and quantifying motor symptoms in PD patients, such as freezing of gait (FOG) and bradykinesia, poses significant therapeutic challenges, particularly in the context of continuous remote patient monitoring.

This study aims to leverage a dataset obtained from smart insoles to evaluate computational approaches focusing on gait assessment. A continuous wavelet transform is employed to transform time series signals into visual representations, departing from conventional methods like recurrent architectures typically utilized in time series analysis.

The results illustrate the effectiveness of the proposed system, achieving an accuracy of 96.5% in analyzing gait variability across three distinct groups (adults, elderly individuals, and PD patients) and a 91% accuracy in evaluating gait symptoms at varying severity levels in PD patients.

7.5.1 Dataset Description

The dataset employed for this research is openly accessible through the Biomedical Informatics Laboratory (BMI) aat: bmi@hmu.gr [15]. This dataset is compiled using wearable insoles that integrate pressure sensors. It encompasses data gathered from three distinct groups, encompassing a total of 29 participants.

7.5.2 Hardware Description

In this research, the dataset utilized is obtained through the use of the Moticon SCIENCE pressure sensor insoles [16], as depicted in Fig. 7.6. These insoles, weighing approximately 80 grams, resemble standard insoles but come equipped with 16

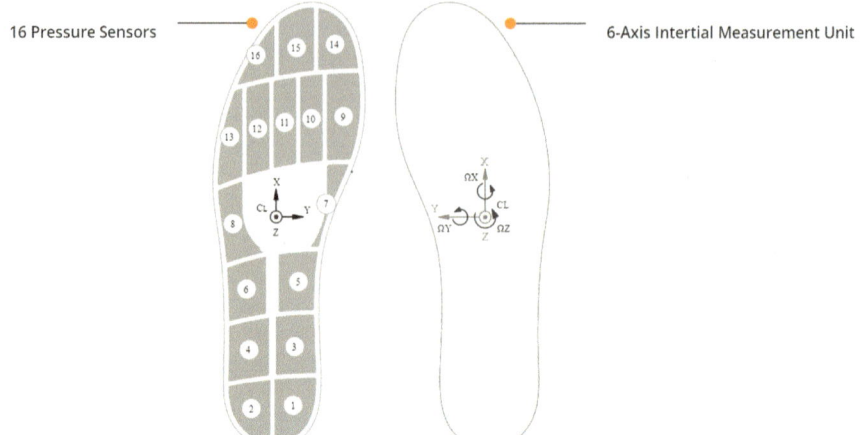

16 Pressure Sensors   6-Axis Intertial Measurement Unit

Fig. 7.6 The framework for sensor insoles and the layout of sensor positions are defined within a standard coordinate framework, as outlined in reference [16]. Notably, the orientation of these coordinate frameworks varies between the left and right sides. The specific placement of the IMU sensor is associated with this coordinate framework. Moreover, distinct orientations of the coordinate system are established for the left and right sides. The sensor data encompasses three spatial dimensions for both acceleration and angular rate information

pressure sensors. The insoles seamlessly integrate power supply, storage, and data transmission components, operating wirelessly. Moreover, they feature a 6-Axis IMU sensor that captures acceleration and angular rate data. Previous studies have validated the functionality and accuracy of these insoles, as evidenced in [17]. Braun et al. [18] assessed their reliability by gathering gait data from 12 healthy subjects on a treadmill at varying speeds. Similarly, [19] conducted trials involving walking, running, and jumping, confirming that these intelligent wearable insoles are suitable for evaluating temporal, force, and balance parameters during diverse gait strides in both clinical and research scenarios. To facilitate the recordings, lightweight and adaptable pairs of shoes were acquired to accommodate the fitted insoles.

A sampling rate of 100 Hz was configured. Each recording yields a file that encompasses a total of 51 features. These include 25 values for the left leg, 25 values for the right leg, and a timestamp.

1. The timestamp (ms)
2. The pressure from 1 to 16 sensors (N/cm^2)
3. The acceleration in the x, y, z axes (g)
4. The angular rate in $w_x, w_y, w_z (dps)$
5. The computed center of pressure in the x,y coordinates (−0.5 . . . +0.5 (related to insole length/width))
6. The total force (N) computed by Moticon.

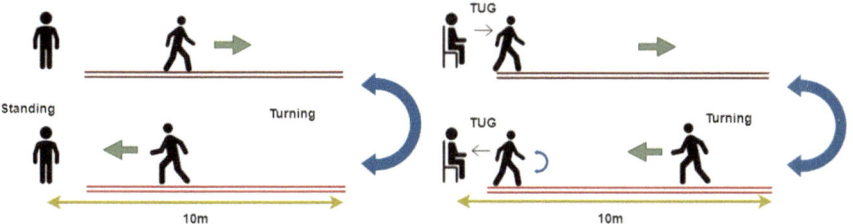

Fig. 7.7 Walking straight test and the timed up and go test

7.5.3 Participants Details

The dataset consists of 29 recordings obtained from participants who have been categorized into three distinct groups, as outlined in Table 7.3. Among these groups, one serves as the control group, comprised of healthy individuals aged between 20 and 59 years. The subsequent group encompasses elderly participants aged 60 years and older. For both of these cohorts, individuals with musculoskeletal or neurological conditions that could potentially impact their gait or balance were excluded from participation. The third group of significant interest is comprised of individuals diagnosed with Parkinson's disease (PD), regardless of their age. All PD subjects adhered to their regular medication schedule. In situations where patients or participants would face challenges in completing all tests, the number and repetitions of tests were adjusted to ensure their comfort and willingness to participate.

An expert neurologist specializing in movement disorders assessed the participants' performance by assigning ratings to four aspects of part III 'Motor examination' of the MDS-UPDRS [20]. These items include item 3.9 "Arising from chair," item 3.10 "Gait," item 3.11 "Freezing of gait," and item 3.14 "Global suddenness of movement" aligning with the employed measurement protocol. In this manner, the neurologist meticulously reviewed video recordings captured by two cameras–one at the end and one at the midpoint of the 10 m course–used during the recording sessions.

Earlier research has demonstrated the feasibility of remotely assessing PD patients, even via video-conference sessions, for part III "Motor examination" of the MDS-UPDRS (excluding item 3.3 "Rigidity" and item 3.12 "Postural stability," which require in-person evaluation). The MDS-UPDRS scores assigned by the neurologist for each participant are presented in Table 7.4.

Experimental Protocol

Numerous research investigations have subsequently pursued various experimental procedures to evaluate attributes of gait, postural stability, and the likelihood of falling among individuals exhibiting either normal or abnormal gait patterns. Gait variability, a measurable characteristic of walking, undergoes changes both in terms

Table 7.4 The MDS-UPDRS rating score for each PD participant

Code name	UPDRS-3.9 Arising from chair	UPDRS-3.10 Gait	UPDRS-3.11 Freezing of gait	UPDRS-3.14 Global spontaneity of movement
PD001	N/A	N/A	N/A	N/A
PD002	0	1	0	1
PD003	4	4	4	4
PD004	1	1	0	1
PD005	3	2	1	3
PD006	0	1	0	1
PD007	1	2	0	2
PD008	4	3	0	3
EL001	0	0	0	0
EL002	1	1	0	1
EL003	1	0	0	0
EL004	1	0	0	0
EL006	0	0	0	0
EL007	1	1	0	1
EL008	0	0	0	0
EL009	0	0	0	0
EL010	0	0	0	0
S001	0	0	0	0
S002	0	0	0	0
S003	0	0	0	0
S004	0	0	0	0
S005	0	0	0	0
S006	0	0	0	0
S007	0	0	0	0
S008	0	0	0	0
S009	0	0	0	0
S010	0	0	0	0
S011	0	0	0	0
S012	0	1	0	0
S013	0	0	0	0

Table 7.5 Activities of Daily Living (ADLS): annotation of smart-insole dataset

Label	Activity	Description
STD	Standing	Standing with subtle movements
STE	Standing eyes closed	Standing with eyes closed
WAL	Walking	Normal walking
WAS	Walking slow	Walking in a slow rhythm
WAF	Walking fast	Walking in a fast rhythm
SCH	Sit on chair	Sitting on a chair
CHU	Chair up	Getting up from a chair
SIT	Sitting	Sitting with subtle movements
TUR	Turning	Turning 180°, in a normal speed at the end of the 10 m aisle
TUS	Turning slow	Turning 180°, in a slow speed at the end of the 10 m aisle
TUF	Turning fast	Turning 180°, in a fast speed at the end of the 10 m aisle

of magnitude and dynamics. The pace of walking, recognized as an increasingly significant physiological factor [21], requires normalization for clinical application, with outcomes carefully organized for clinical research purposes [22].

The majority of these experimental protocols involve trials encompassing several steps along a straight path and at varying velocities. These trials also include walking on inclined surfaces and staircases. In the case of individuals with Parkinson's disease (PwPD), three primary tests are frequently conducted: (1) the Timed Up and Go test (TUG test) [23–25], where subjects rise from a seated position, walk, and then return to sit on a chair; (2) walking in a corridor with obstacles [26, 27], and (3) the Dual-Task test, where participants walk while simultaneously engaging in a secondary activity such as mental arithmetic, conversation, object manipulation, etc. [28, 29]. Given the significance of these trials, the smart insoles dataset incorporates the Walking Straight and Turn test as well as a modified version of the Timed Up and Go test, depicted in Fig. 7.7. The labeling of the dataset was carried out through a clarifying process. The initial level of Activity of Daily Living (ADL) elucidation comprised 12 distinct labels (Table 7.5), delineating the sequence of activities undertaken by participants during the tests.

7.6 Materials and Methods

The methodological approach of the proposed system is elucidated in Fig. 7.8. The data originating from wearable insoles takes the form of time series data produced

Fig. 7.8 The method of building the gait analysis model

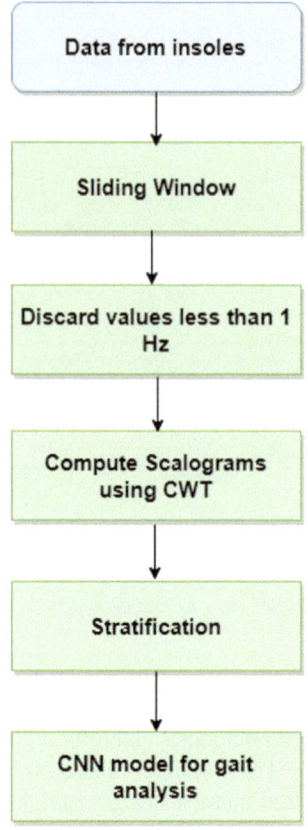

by pressure sensors. Initially, these raw signals undergo preprocessing and filtering procedures. Subsequently, a sliding window of 3 s is employed to generate scalograms via continuous wavelet transform (CWT). This transformation converts the time series data into images, which are subsequently subjected to analysis to detect gait anomalies and estimate the severity of Parkinson's disease (PD) symptoms. Stratification is applied, and the analysis is performed using a deep learning convolutional neural network model.

7.6.1   Continuous Wavelet Transform (CWT)

The effectiveness of the CWT method has been established due to its ability to capture both temporal and frequency characteristics. Over recent years, numerous research endeavors have employed either Fourier transform or short-time Fourier transform to extract features for PD motor symptoms, originating from signals related to lower

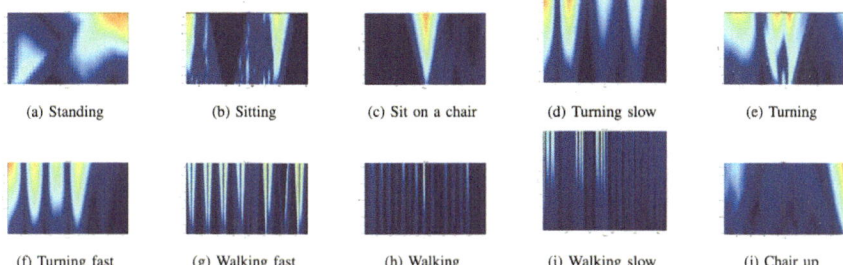

Fig. 7.9 Scalograms of different motor tasks performed by one of the PD patients

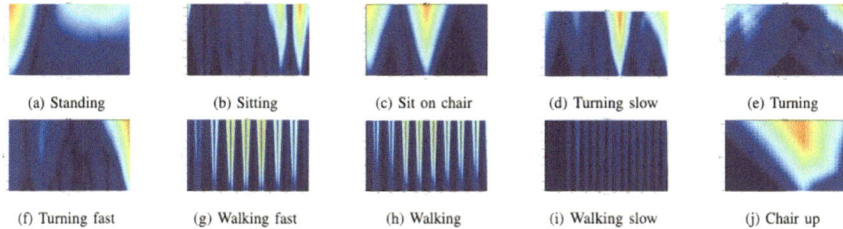

Fig. 7.10 Scalograms of different motor tasks performed by one of the subject belonging to the elderly cohort

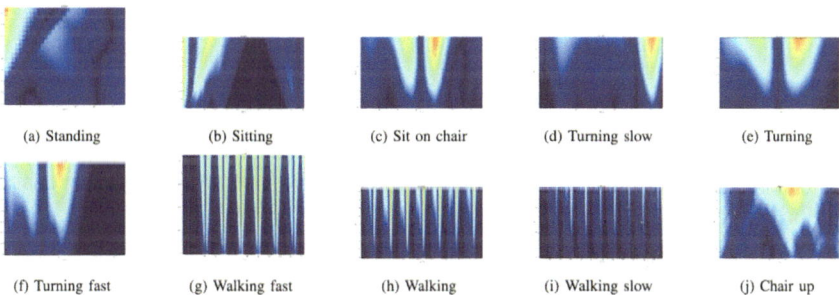

Fig. 7.11 Scalograms of different motor tasks performed by one of the subject belonging to the adult cohort

body motion or upper limb motion. Nonetheless, both of these methods struggle to pinpoint the precise location of an event. As a solution, an extensive array of features is extracted. However, as the quantity of features increases, energy consumption and latency issues begin to impact data storage, event processing, and analysis.

The CWT of a signal is represented by Eq. 7.4.

$$CWT(a, b) = \langle f, \Psi_{a,b} \rangle = 1/\sqrt{a} \int_{-\infty}^{\infty} f(t).\Psi * (t - b/a)dt \qquad (7.4)$$

Here Ψ addresses the wavelet mother function, which is a template basis function of limited length, zero mean and variable recurrence content, an and b signify the dilatation (or scale) and moving (or shifting) factors (which decide how much the mother wavelet is scaled and translated), CWT (a, b) addresses the wavelet coefficients and $*$ is the complex conjugate operator. In our case, the 'Haar' wavelet has been used. As our dataset is already filtered out and labeled, the haar wavelet type suits perfectly to our problem.

Scalograms produced through CWT are depicted in Figs. 7.9, 7.10, and 7.11. The dissimilarities observed in these scalograms elucidate the alterations in gait attributes among various participant groups. The process of generating scalograms entails constructing a sliding window that captures samples of consistent activities, thereby generating scalograms specific to each task.

During the transformation of time series data into images, an essential consideration was to ensure that the frequency content remained below 1 Hz. TThe distinctive colors observed in the scalograms convey the variations in gait variability across all participant cohorts. The cumulative count of generated scalograms approximates 7500 images.

Deep learning ConvNet model

The primary goal of this study is to effectively categorize the scalograms constructed using CWT [30, 31] into distinct stages of Parkinson's disease (PD) patients, as well as to accurately diagnose gait attributes within all participant cohorts. In this research endeavor, the ConvNet architecture was employed for experimentation, with variations in weights to achieve optimal outcomes. The initial step involves resizing the input scalograms to dimensions of $227 \times 227 \times 3$. These dimensions correspond to the width, height, and three color channels, representing the image's depth. Subsequently, these scalograms are fed into the convolutional layer input, where a sequence of convolutional filters is applied to identify specific features within the images. This is followed by ReLU and max pooling layers, repeated convolution and max pooling steps, and ultimately, three additional convolution layers followed by max pooling. The architecture culminates in fully connected layers.

The results following the training and testing of scalograms are illustrated in Fig. 7.12. The model is trained using a 70/30 split of training and testing data. Evaluation metrics utilized in this study include the confusion matrix, a tool that facilitates the visualization of classification performance, as depicted in Fig. 7.12. The confusion matrix enables the computation of various metrics, including accuracy, misclassification, precision, sensitivity, and specificity. In the figure, correct predictions are denoted by green boxes, while incorrect predictions are represented by red ones.

This study presents an innovative solution for clinically evaluating gait variability among individuals. The developed system aids medical professionals in making informed decisions during the initial assessment of elderly individuals or patients with PD, as well as during the monitoring of their progress and the effects of treatments. Instead of extracting an extensive array of temporal or spectral features, the

Fig. 7.12 a represents confusion matrix of gait variability analysis and **b** confusion matrix for severity analysis

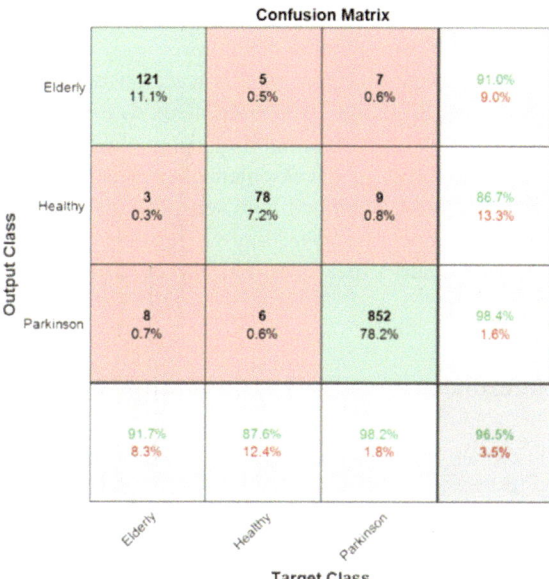

(a) Confusion matrix of gait variability analysis

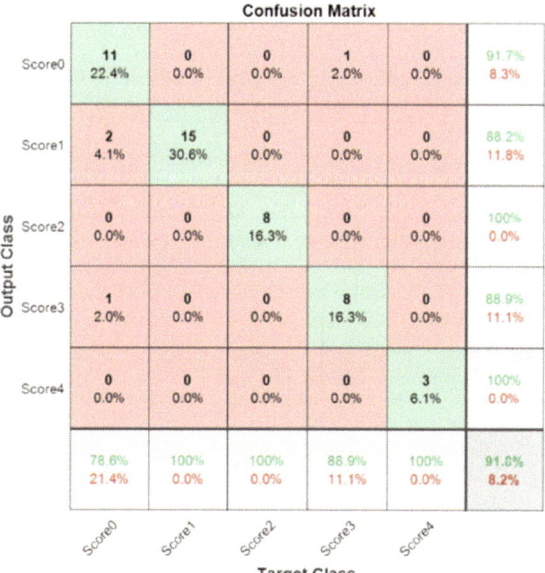

(b) Confusion matrix for severity analysis

system generates scalograms using the CWT, and by processing them through a CNN model, it yields promising outcomes.

The primary objective of this research is to introduce a new approach to gait assessment, utilizing CWT-based methods to address the analysis of idiopathic PD severity levels and gait variability in age-matched cohorts. Moving forward, a future prospect involves the development of an eHealth platform centered around a compact wearable device equipped with sensors capable of capturing crucial motor signals from both upper and lower limbs. This device would feature wireless connectivity, enhanced security measures, and improved power efficiency.

References

1. Gaßner, H., Jensen, D., Marxreiter, F., Kletsch, A., Bohlen, S., Schubert, R., Muratori, L., Eskofier, B., Klucken, J., Winkler, J. & Others Gait variability as digital biomarker of disease severity in Huntington's disease. *Journal Of Neurology*. pp. 1–8 (2020)
2. Montero-Odasso, M. & Camicioli, R. Falls and Cognition in Older Persons: Fundamentals, Assessment and Therapeutic Options. (Springer Nature,2019)
3. Wood, B., Bilclough, J., Bowron, A. & Walker, R. Incidence and prediction of falls in Parkinson's disease: a prospective multidisciplinary study. *Journal Of Neurology, Neurosurgery & Psychiatry*. **72**, 721–725 (2002)
4. Hausdorff, J., Cudkowicz, M., Firtion, R., Wei, J. & Goldberger, A. Gait variability and basal ganglia disorders: stride-to-stride variations of gait cycle timing in Parkinson's disease and Huntington's disease. *Movement Disorders*. **13**, 428–437 (1998)
5. Yacchirema, D., Puga, J., Palau, C. & Esteve, M. Fall detection system for elderly people using IoT and ensemble machine learning algorithm. *Personal And Ubiquitous Computing*. **23**, 801–817 (2019)
6. Chandra, I., Sivakumar, N., Gokulnath, C. & Parthasarathy, P. IoT based fall detection and ambient assisted system for the elderly. *Cluster Computing*. **22**, 2517–2525 (2019)
7. Hussain, F., Umair, M., Haq, M., Pires, I., Valente, T., Garcia, N. & Pombo, N. An Efficient Machine Learning-based Elderly Fall Detection Algorithm. ArXiv Preprint ArXiv:1911.11976. (2019)
8. Nandy, A. Statistical methods for analysis of parkinson's disease gait pattern and classification. *Multimedia Tools And Applications*. **78**, 19697–19734 (2019)
9. Joshi, D., Khajuria, A. & Joshi, P. An automatic non-invasive method for Parkinson's disease classification. *Computer Methods And Programs In Biomedicine*. **145** pp. 135–145 (2017)
10. Wahid, F., Begg, R., Hass, C., Halgamuge, S. & Ackland, D. Classification of Parkinson's disease gait using spatial-temporal gait features. *IEEE Journal Of Biomedical And Health Informatics*. **19**, 1794–1802 (2015)
11. Goldberger, A., L. Amaral, L. Glass, J. Hausdorff, P. C. Ivanov, R. Mark, J. E. Mietus, G. B. Moody, C. K. Peng, and H. E. Stanley PhysioBank, PhysioToolkit, and PhysioNet: Components of a new research resource for complex physiologic signals, Circulation [Online]. 101 (23), pp. e215–e220. (2000)
12. Hausdorff, J., Mitchell, S., Firtion, R., Peng, C., Cudkowicz, M., Wei, J. & Goldberger, A. Altered fractal dynamics of gait: reduced stride-interval correlations with aging and Huntington's disease. *Journal Of Applied Physiology*. **82**, 262–269 (1997)
13. Bryce, R. & Sprague, K. Revisiting detrended fluctuation analysis. *Scientific Reports*. **2**, 1–6 (2012)
14. Yue, J., Zhao, X. & Shang, P. Effect of trends on detrended fluctuation analysis of precipitation series. *Mathematical Problems In Engineering*. **2010** (2010)

15. BMI Lab, *The Smart-Insole Dataset*, https://bmi.hmu.gr/the-smart-insole-dataset/ [Accessed September 4, 2023]

16. *Moticon Science*, "Sensor Insoles for Research," https://www.moticon.de/ [Accessed September 4, 2023].

17. T. P. Kakarla et al., "Accuracy enhancement of total force by capacitive insoles," in *2019 IEEE International Symposium on Medical Measurements and Applications (MeMeA)*, pp. 1–6, 2019.

18. B. J. Braun et al., "Validation and reliability testing of a new, fully integrated gait analysis insole," *Journal of foot and ankle research*, vol. 8, no. 1, pp. 1–7, 2015.

19. T. Stöggl and A. Martiner, "Validation of Moticon's OpenGo sensor insoles during gait, jumps, balance and cross-country skiing specific imitation movements," *Journal of sports sciences*, vol. 35, no. 2, pp. 196–206, 2017.

20. C. G. Goetz et al., "Movement Disorder Society-sponsored revision of the Unified Parkinson's Disease Rating Scale (MDS-UPDRS): scale presentation and clinimetric testing results," *Movement disorders: official journal of the Movement Disorder Society*, vol. 23, no. 15, pp. 2129–2170, 2008.

21. A. Middleton, S. L. Fritz, and M. Lusardi, "Walking speed: the functional vital sign," *Journal of aging and physical activity*, vol. 23, no. 2, pp. 314–322, 2015.

22. J. E. Graham, G. V. Ostir, Y. -F. Kuo, S. R. Fisher, and K. J. Ottenbacher, "Relationship between test methodology and mean velocity in timed walk tests: a review," *Archives of physical medicine and rehabilitation*, vol. 89, no. 5, pp. 865–872, 2008.

23. S. Morris, M. E. Morris, and R. Iansek, "Reliability of measurements obtained with the Timed "Up & Go" test in people with Parkinson disease," *Physical therapy*, vol. 81, no. 2, pp. 810–818, 2001.

24. C. M. Campbell, J. L. Rowse, M. A. Ciol, and A. Shumway-Cook, "The effect of cognitive demand on timed up and go performance in older adults with and without Parkinson disease," *Journal of Neurologic Physical Therapy*, vol. 27, no. 1, pp. 2–7, 2003.

25. M. Scicchitano and B. Rocchi, "Quantitative evaluation of instrumented time up and go test in subjects with Parkinson disease: the evaluation of a new rehabilitative treatment," Italy, 2018.

26. Steven T. Moore, Don A. Yungher, Tiffany R. Morris, Valentina Dilda, Hamish G. MacDougall, James M. Shine, Sharon L. Naismith, Simon JG. Lewis, *Autonomous identification of freezing of gait in Parkinson's disease from lower-body segmental accelerometry*, Journal of Neuroengineering and Rehabilitation, vol. 10, no. 1, pp. 1–11, 2013.

27. Yaejin Moon, Douglas A. Wajda, Robert W. Motl, Jacob J. Sosnoff, *Stride-time variability and fall risk in persons with multiple sclerosis*, Multiple Sclerosis International, vol. 2015, pp. 1–6, 2015.

28. A. Z. da Silva and V. L. Israel, "Effects of dual-task aquatic exercises on functional mobility, balance and gait of individuals with Parkinson's disease: A randomized clinical trial with a 3-month follow-up," *Complementary Therapies in Medicine*, vol. 42, pp. 119–124, 2019.

29. Roisin C. Vance, Dan G. Healy, Rose Galvin, Helen P. French, *Dual tasking with the timed "up & go" test improves detection of risk of falls in people with Parkinson disease*, Physical Therapy, vol. 95, no. 1, pp. 95–102, 2015.

30. N. Ji, H. Zhou, K. Guo, O. W. Samuel, Z. Huang, L. Xu, and G. Li, "Appropriate mother wavelets for continuous gait event detection based on time-frequency analysis for hemiplegic and healthy individuals," *Sensors*, vol. 19, no. 16, p. 3462, 2019.

31. M. Alafeef and M. Fraiwan, "On the diagnosis of idiopathic Parkinson's disease using continuous wavelet transform complex plot," *Journal of Ambient Intelligence and Humanized Computing*, vol. 10, no. 7, pp. 2805–2815, 2019.

Chapter 8
Conclusion and Prospects for Further Development

Abstract This concluding chapter encapsulates the key findings and contributions of the research presented in this book. It commences by highlighting the transformative therapeutic advancements that have converted PD from a life-threatening condition into a manageable disease. Nevertheless, the intricate and progressive nature of PD continues to pose challenges for its effective management and the enhancement of patients' quality of life. The chapter accentuates the originality of the research work, centering on the development of the A-WEAR bracelet as a cost-effective and tailored wearable device for PD assessment. A comprehensive comparison is drawn between the A-WEAR bracelet and existing motion data collection devices, accentuating the advantages of the A-WEAR bracelet in terms of cost, capabilities, and integration with a cloud platform. Furthermore, the chapter scrutinizes the validation and support offered to prevailing theories and models in the field of PD monitoring. It highlights the creation of an objective monitoring system for assessing PD symptoms, which employs meticulous preprocessing, feature extraction, and model evaluation techniques.

8.1 Originality of Research Work

Over the course of more than two centuries, PD has been a subject of medical research. During this time, therapeutic advancements have transformed it from a fatal condition to a manageable disease with varying degrees of long-term effectiveness. A range of approaches, including pharmacological and non-pharmacological interventions like surgeries and multidisciplinary care, have become available. However, despite these treatments, the complex and diverse nature of PD continues to progress, ultimately leading to a significant decline in quality of life. Thus, we contend that current medical research has not yet provided practical tools to PD patients for effectively managing the intricacies of their condition on a daily basis, tailored to their individual needs and enabling efficient self-care.

This book presents the utilization of wearable technology in the form of an eHealth system as a means to enhance self-care, assess motor activities, and recommend appropriate treatments in PD. Each component of the system, from the prototype to the cloud platform and the functioning of the DL approach within the cloud, has been developed taking into account all potential limitations and opportunities.

The work expounded in this book represents a substantial and noteworthy contribution to the accumulated state-of-the-art in the domain of automatic monitoring of Parkinson's disease (PD) patients. We have proposed a robust and sophisticated solution, in the form of a cutting-edge wearable device, for the comprehensive assessment of individuals affected by PD. As elucidated in Chap. 3, while there exist numerous wearable devices for motion data collection and monitoring, they are invariably accompanied by inherent limitations. For instance, popular devices like Fitbit, Garmin, or Apple watches equipped with inertial sensors primarily focus on tracking step counts or heart rates for fitness purposes and are not specifically designed to cater to the unique demands of PD patients. Similarly, the data analyzed in the research segment described in Chap. 4, was collected using a Shimmer3 device. Due to the unprecedented COVID-19 pandemic, it was impractical to construct a dataset directly from PD patients, thus necessitating the utilization of data from the Shimmer unit for comparative purposes. In Chap. 4, we provided a thorough comparison between the data collected from our proposed bracelet and the data obtained from the Shimmer3 device.

The rationale behind developing the A-WEAR bracelet, despite the existence of a device named Shimmer for motion data collection, can be attributed to several decisive factors. Firstly, the Shimmer3 device incurs a substantial cost of up to 430 Euros, while our bracelet offers a significantly more economical alternative at a mere 50 Euros. Furthermore, the Shimmer3 device is primarily designed to collect motion data for preclinical studies, lacking the intricate capabilities required for the specific needs of PD patients. In contrast, our A-WEAR bracelet not only facilitates data collection but also encompasses advanced analytical features and seamless integration with a cloud platform, enabling continuous and tailored assessment of PD patients. Moreover, our bracelet offers the distinctive advantage of customizable sampling frequency and time spectrum of data collection, a feature absent in both the Shimmer3 device and other commercially available wearable devices presently accessible in the market.

In addition to the aforementioned contributions, this book also provides substantial validation and support for prevailing theories, models, and interpretations in the field. As outlined in section Chap. 3, several researchers resort to employing multiple sensor nodes on patients for data analysis or restrict their data collection to a limited timeframe during specific exercises. Furthermore, a significant number of studies overlook the critical consideration of accurate tremor severity distribution. In Chap. 4, we address these issues by developing an objective monitoring system that effectively and automatically assesses PD symptoms, akin to the well-established Unified Parkinson's Disease Rating Scale (UPDRS). The data obtained from the bracelet is subjected to meticulous preprocessing and rigorous feature extraction. Leveraging the FeatureWiz Python library, we employ an automated feature selection process, significantly reducing input variables and eliminating noise from the data. To optimize model performance and achieve precise estimation, we adopt rigorous cross-validation techniques and employ resampling methodologies, as evidenced by the comprehensive tests. Unlike prior studies expounded upon in Chap. 4, our proposed model is evaluated not merely based on accuracy, precision, sensitivity, and specificity, but also by leveraging metrics such as F1-score, Gmean, and IBAα, thus elevating the scientific rigor and depth of our evaluation framework.

8.2 Future Work

This section delves into the primary avenues for prospective research following the completion of this book.

1. Develop and evaluate a functional prototype of a wearable device, utilizing the insights presented in Chap. 3, by incorporating the practical experiences of both PD patients and medical experts. This iterative process aims to ensure broad acceptance and effective implementation of the smart eHealth system for monitoring and assessing individuals with PD. This endeavor may lead to improvements in the functionality, comfort, and aesthetics of the wearable device.
2. In this research investigation, the data is subjected to offline processing to evaluate the severity of PD tremors. Hence, it would be captivating to engage PD patients directly in the data collection and interpretation phase, while utilizing our A-WEAR wristband for uninterrupted remote monitoring.
3. Use of data centric approaches rather than model centric ones which focus on data processing in terms of labeling quality, novel argumentation schemes
4. Enhancements to the user-friendly interface we have developed for patients and physicians could prove beneficial in simplifying the method for estimating tremor severity. For instance, incorporating voice-overs and instructional videos can assist in training patients on data acquisition and other related tasks. Furthermore, it would be advantageous to devise a system that allows physicians to comprehensively evaluate and communicate data analysis findings, akin to existing grading systems, facilitating effective communication and assessment.
5. Chapter 3 introduces our proposed framework that focuses on analyzing tremors based on accelerometer signals. In future research, we aim to expand this framework to explore other key symptoms, such as FoG, bradykinesia, or gait variability. This exploration will involve investigating various DL techniques, utilizing different window sizes and overlaps, to effectively analyze and capture these symptoms.
6. This book solely utilizes accelerometer and gyroscope signals for analysis. However, future research endeavors could consider incorporating additional signals, such as electromyography (EMG), or exploring the combined use of multiple signals. This would enable a more comprehensive assessment of tremor direction, in addition to magnitude, enhancing the overall understanding of Parkinson's disease-related tremors.

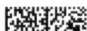

7. Given the findings made in this book, it is worth exploring the application of wearables and smart monitoring systems to other categories of patients affected by NCDs.